THE WAY OF
TEA

THE WAY OF
TEA

THE SUBLIME ART OF ORIENTAL TEA DRINKING

MASTER LAM KAM CHUEN
with **LAM KAI SIN** *and* **LAM TIN YU**

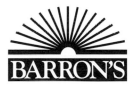

First edition for the United States and Canada published 2002 by Barron's Educational Series, Inc.

All inquiries should be addressed to:
Barron's Educational Series, Inc.
250 Wireless Boulevard
Hauppauge, New York 11788
http://www.barronseduc.com

Library of Congress Catalog Card No. 2001087436
International Standard Book No. 0-7641-1968-0

Printed in Singapore

9 8 7 6 5 4 3 2 1

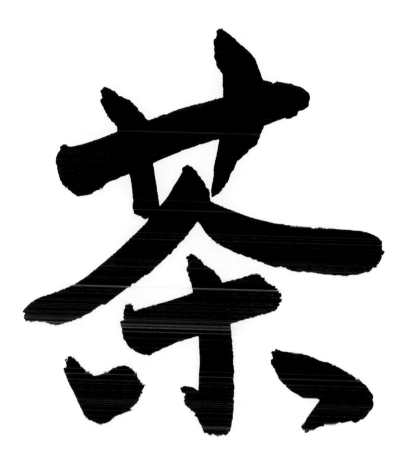

Ch'a, or tea

Contents

8–11 Introduction

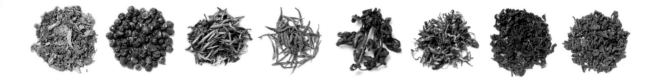

PART ONE
Tea Story
12–37

The Discovery of Tea
The Development of Tea in China
Tea-drinking Customs in China
The Spread of Tea from China

PART TWO
Cultivating Tea
38–71

Tea Plants and Their Varieties
Picking the Tea Leaves
Tea Processing Through the Ages
Monkey-picked Tea
White Teas
Yellow Teas
Light Green Teas
Green Teas
Red Teas
Black Teas
Flower Teas

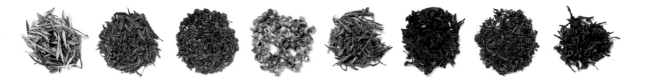

PART THREE
Tea Time
72–111

Water, the Mother of Tea
Heating the Water
Teapots, the Father of Tea
Storing Tea Leaves
The Art of Tea Making
Kung Fu Tea

PART FOUR
Healing Teas
112–139

A Culture of Health
Introducing the Healing Teas
Cautions and Uses of Tea

140 About the Authors
141 Acknowledgments
142–143 Index

"…Tea leaves are the product,
the embodiment of the three elements —
Heaven, Earth and Man…
by Heaven we mean the climate and the weather…
by Earth we mean soil fertility…
Man refers to the process, the work of
making tea from the leaves."

Introduction

Tea to the Chinese is as wine to Westerners: an endless source of romance and inspiration, with its subtly changing color, aroma, and taste. There are many different kinds of tea to suit individual and social tastes, each one able to refresh the palate, restore the spirits, and help cure and prevent minor ailments. Since its discovery in China thousands of years ago, peasant farmers have lovingly tended tea plants, or *Camellia sinensis*, and harvested and processed their leaves. Tea was a drink for emperors and peasants alike, so although the highest quality leaves were reserved for the sophisticated palates of emperors and their courtiers, everybody enjoyed the variety and healing properties of tea. Tea folklore has been passed down through generations, preserving stories of how the different tea plants were discovered and named.

A tea culture is born

The Chinese were quick to recognize the many benefits of tea and by the Han Dynasty (206 B.C.–A.D. 221) were conducting extensive research into this ancient drink. Generation after generation studied where and how tea grew, which soil was best, which climate the most clement, which leaves to pick and when to harvest them, as well as how to handle, treat, and preserve the leaves. Out of this painstaking research grew their profound knowledge of tea cultivation and processing. The imperial courts of the Tang, Sung, and Ming Dynasties spearheaded the demand for tea and played a large part in establising tea-drinking customs. As the thirst for tea grew, emperors encouraged tea masters to create new teas with a variety of tastes and flavors. Thus the Chinese tradition of tea was born.

The global market

As the news of this remarkable drink spread around the world, everyone wanted to share in its delights, each nation establishing its own tea traditions and discovering a place for tea in its own social rituals. Needless to say, when the time came, the British (in India) and the Dutch (in Indonesia) wanted to grow the crop and reap the rich rewards of exporting it for themselves. However, they lacked the expertise, craftsmanship, and intimate knowledge held only by the Chinese tea masters. By diplomacy of the most varied kind, both the British and Dutch managed to persuade the Chinese to reveal their secrets and went on to establish the tea plantations that have since dominated the world.

In order to satisfy the enormous thirst of the global market, the Dutch and British plantations turned to machinery in the 19th century to manufacture their teas. In the process they turned what was once an individually handcrafted beverage into a rather bland, mass-produced, blended drink. These teas are expected to taste the same year after year, yet still claim to be selected, handpicked, and of the finest quality.

Meanwhile the Chinese have persevered with creating their rich variety of teas using their traditional, organic, and manual methods. It is said that China produces over 10,000 teas each year, with names that seem baffling to all but the connoisseur. Yet the diversity of teas from China means that everyone has a chance to discover the flavors and tastes they prefer and therefore find a tea to suit their temperament and constitution, as well as satisfy their palate and social needs.

The six types of tea

This book differs from many others because it focuses on six types of tea, namely green, light green, yellow, red, white, and black teas. The first four are so-called because of the color of the brew they make, while white teas have earned their name from their whitened leaves. Black teas are named after the color of their taste — a bitterness that must be sampled to be believed. In the West, even though the tea leaves look black, most people drink red tea, either loose or in standard tea bags.

Because of the current consumer concerns surrounding the safety of mass-produced, manufactured foods, many large tea plantations are now marketing organic tea. However, Master Lam is doubtful whether true organic growing can work on such a large scale, for where monoculture prevails it is hard to control pests and diseases without using damaging chemicals.

This book is a celebration of the Chinese way of tea, where the sensitive touch of the tea maker's fingertips can mean the difference between a good quality tea and an ordinary one. Such intricacies of processing, not to mention traditions of brewing and serving tea, have been passed down from generation to generation and are still very much alive today. The Chinese way of tea is an art that combines the appreciation of the remarkable tastes, flavors, and healing properties of the many different teas with respect for the tea and its drinkers.

Silk scroll dating from the Tang Dynasty (A.D. 618–907)
when tea drinking was becoming increasingly fashionable.
The woman on the left holds a pipa, a stringed instrument from northwest China that is similar to a mandolin.
The woman to her right carries a tray of tea bowls.

PART ONE

Tea Story

The Discovery of Tea 14–15

The Development of Tea in China 16–21

Tea-drinking Customs in China 22–23

The Spread of Tea from China 24–37

13

The Discovery of Tea

Nobody knows when tea was discovered in China, although as a mark of respect it is traditionally ascribed to the mythical Chinese emperor Shên Nung. Shên Nung ruled for 17 generations before 2700 B.C. and is the father of Chinese medicine. He is famous for his knowledge of the medicinal properties of herbs and plants and traditionally venerated by apothecaries.

There are two versions of how Shên Nung discovered tea. The first tells how Shên Nung was tasting different kinds of plants when he suddenly felt very sick: his mouth became dry, his tongue uncomfortable, and he felt hot. He searched around for a cure and noticed some leaves on the ground that had fallen from a nearby tree. Out of habit and curiosity he picked them up and tasted them. Although bitter they had a pleasant fragrance and afterward he felt better. He collected more leaves from the same tree and took them home with him to investigate their properties.

The second version describes how one day Shên Nung, tired from his work, made a fire below a tree to heat some water. Some leaves from the tree fell into his pot of water, which he then tasted. It was at once bitter and sweet, and he drank the entire pot. Afterward he felt refreshed and more awake. He realized that he had found a new and useful herb and decided to investigate it further. When he tasted the tea it is said that Shên Nung felt a warmth passing through him, like a device testing every part of his body. This is why tea was named "ch'a," the same word as the Chinese character meaning to test, check, or investigate. Later it was given a new character, also pronounced "ch'a," which shows wood at the bottom, flowers and grass at the top, and a man between the two. This is symbolic of how tea can help bring humankind into balance with nature.

After Shên Nung's discovery the Chinese studied tea leaves and began to cultivate them. The earliest records of tea harvesting date from around 2000 B.C. when tea drinking was already well established. In the ancient medical text, *The Yellow Emperor's Classic of Internal Medicine*, the court physician speaks to the great emperor Huang Ti of the tea trees in the cold region of Szechuan. There the trees grew very tall and straight:

"Bittert'u is called ch'a, hsuan and yu. It grows in winter in the valleys by the streams, and on the hills of Ichow [in the province of Szechuan], and does not perish in severe winter. It is gathered on the third day of the third month [in April] and then dried."

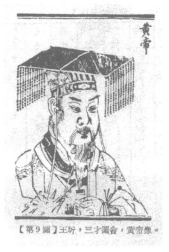

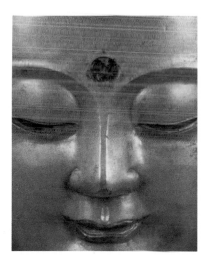

Above This woodcut is a rare portrait of the Yellow Emperor, Huang Ti.

Left A page from an old edition of The Yellow Emperor's Classic of Internal Medicine.

Bodhidharma's eyelids

Although Shén Nung is traditionally associated with the discovery of tea, there is another story surrounding Bodhidharma, an Indian Buddhist monk. He lived around the 6th century A.D. and is considered the father of Zen Buddhism. According to folklore, Bodhidharma fell asleep during a seven-year-long meditation. When he awoke he was very angry with himself and, in order to prevent it from happening again, cut off his eyelids. It is said that where they fell two tea plants grew.

The Development of Tea in China

There is a Chinese household saying that when you leave your bedroom in the morning there are seven things essential to your life, namely firewood, rice, oil, salt, spicy sauce, vinegar, and tea. However, it was some time before tea was regarded as an everyday beverage or even as a luxury item; indeed, it was used predominantly for medicinal purposes and in *Pen Ts'ao Ching*, an early dictionary of Chinese herbs dating from the Tang Dynasty, it is classified as a bitter herb.

The refreshing properties of tea began to eclipse its medicinal uses during the Chow Dynasty. At this time kings used to drink a crude brew of tea, although it was not very popular as it had an extremely bitter taste. By the Han Dynasty (206 B.C.–A.D. 221) the Chinese had refined their methods of collecting and preparing leaves from wild tea plants. Tea was a more palatable beverage and was much sought after by royal subjects. One day at a royal banquet the king offered wine to all his subjects. However, one of them refused, saying wine made him easily drunk. From this time on whenever the king served wine at his banquets he gave this man tea. The same king helped spread the reputation of tea still further when he presented tea to his subjects as gifts. By the period of the Three Kingdoms (A.D. 221–277) tea had replaced wine at banquets, as people preferred the refreshing properties of tea to the intoxicating effects of wine.

Tea became increasingly fashionable toward the end of the Tang Dynasty (A.D. 618–907) and reached its peak, known as the Golden Age of Tea, during the Sung Dynasty (A.D. 960–1279). Slowly a tea-drinking tradition was born that was to become an integral part of Chinese culture. Different regions evolved their own tea customs, for example how they brewed, served, and drank their tea, as well as the variety of tea plants they grew. This gave rise to a rich and diverse tea-drinking culture throughout China.

Lo Yu, an important but eccentric scholar, was the leading authority on tea during the 8th century and around A.D. 780 wrote the first authoritative book on tea called *Ch'a Ching*. He named any beverage made from the tea plant "ch'a" regardless of the preparation or whether it was unfermented, semi-fermented, or fermented, as until this time they had had different names. According to Lo Yu there were already "a thousand and ten thousand teas." *Ch'a Ching* contains detailed information about tea plants, the different varieties, the ways of processing and brewing tea, tea-drinking customs and traditions, and where to find the purest waters for tea making.

TEA CHRONOLOGY

Circa 2700 B.C.
The mythical Chinese Emperor Shên Nung discovers tea.

206 B.C.–A.D. 221 Han Dynasty
Improvements in methods of collecting tea leaves and brewing attract the attention of royal subjects.

A.D. 221–277 Three Kingdoms
Tea replaces wine at Chinese imperial banquets.

A.D. 618–907 Tang Dynasty
Tea becomes the national drink in China.

A.D. 705 The monk Dengyo Daishi takes tea to Japan.

A.D. 780 Lo Yu, the patron saint of tea, publishes *Ch'a Ching*, a three-volume work on the history, cultivation, and preparation of tea.

A.D. 960–1279 Sung Dynasty
Golden Age of Tea. Tea reaches the peak of fashion.

1191 The Buddhist monk Yesai revives the cultivation of tea in Japan and goes on to publish the first tea book in Japan.

1368–1644 Ming Dynasty
China exports shiploads of porcelain teapots and wooden chests of tea to Portugal, Holland, and England. The Chinese also import silver teapots from Europe: European potteries are unable to produce ceramic teapots as fine, heat resistant, and strong as chinaware.

1610 The Dutch East India Company brings Chinese tea to Europe.

1618 Tea reaches Russia. The Chinese embassy in Moscow gives chests of tea to Tsar Alexis, initiating a trade of camel caravans that traveled over 11,000 miles between China and Russia and took almost a year and a half to complete the journey.

1644–1911 Ching Dynasty
Toward the end of the Ching Dynasty European tea importers, such as the East India companies, establish their own plantations in colonies in India, Ceylon, and Indonesia.

1648 Tea reaches Paris.

Circa 1650 Tea reaches England and America.

1669 The British East India Company imports Chinese tea to London.

1810 Tea cultivation in Formosa, now Taiwan, is started by the Chinese.

1823–1824 Tea is discovered growing indigenously near Rangpur in Assam by Major Robert Bruce and his brother, Charles. This discovery lays the foundations for the Indian tea industry.

1832–1833 The founder and father of tea in Indonesia, the Dutchman J. I. L. L. Jacobson, brings back from China around seven million tea seeds and 15 Chinese planters, as well as tea makers and box makers. The Chinese authorities are so angry they put a price on his head.

1869 Coffee blight strikes the enormously productive coffee plantations in Ceylon, which are finally wiped out during the infestation of 1877–1878. This triggered a rush back into tea.

1900 The final camel caravan transporting tea to Russia leaves Beijing (Peking), just before the Trans-Siberian Railway is completed.

1904 Richard Blechynden invents iced tea at the Worlds Fair in St. Louis.

1908 Thomas Sullivan, a tea merchant from New York, invents the tea bag.

1911 Chinese Republic established after overthrowing the Manchu Dynasty.

1949 People's Republic of China founded.

1997–1999 The average annual production of dried tea leaves in the world is approximately 3.3 million tons. Around 28 percent comes from India, almost 23 percent from China, almost 10 percent from Sri Lanka, 8 percent from Kenya, and 5 percent from Indonesia. The remainder comes from countries such as Turkey, Japan, Iran, and Argentina.

The story of Lo Yu, the tea scholar

Lo Yu was born in A.D. 733 and died in A.D. 804. Nothing is known about his family background, as he was abandoned as a baby. He was found by a Buddhist monk who was walking around a lake. The monk saw wild geese circling in the air above lots of tall reeds and, looking closer, saw a small baby sitting among the reeds while being fed by the geese. When the monk lifted up the boy the geese started attacking him, but he managed to escape with him back to the monastery. At first the monk called him Fei Sing, meaning "shooting star," but that made the baby cry, as did all the other names he tried. One day the monk called him Lo Yu, and the baby blinked but didn't cry. "Lo" means earth and "Yu" means feather, so the name tells the story of Lo Yu's past: he arrived from nowhere like a feather falling from the sky and landing on the ground.

As a boy Lo Yu was very clever, writing poetry by the time he was nine. He also developed a love of tea. However, he did not enjoy the monastic way of life and ran away when he was 12. Fortunately, he met people who recognized his talents and he was able to study literature. He also began to recognize the healing properties of tea. By the time he was 21, Lo Yu decided he would devote himself to studying tea and began to collect and research it. By A.D. 764 he had written his first draft of the famous *Ch'a Ching* and in A.D. 780 the first edition was published. *Ch'a Ching* was immediately recognized as an encyclopedia of tea, as other books on tea simply did not compare to the details and specifications of Lo Yu's work. Thus *Ch'a Ching* became a reference for later works on tea.

Initially, *Ch'a Ching* was only well known among tea lovers, although its reputation eventually spread outside China. On one occasion a Muslim emissary was sent to emperor Tang to obtain a copy: the Muslim was to offer 1,000 battle horses in exchange for a copy of *Ch'a Ching*. The Chinese emperor had not heard of the book but spent a long time looking for it. Eventually he found a copy for the emissary to take home and as a result *Ch'a Ching* was translated into many languages and became well known throughout the world. Impressed by the Muslim interest, the emperor also read the book and recognized the talent of its author. He sent subjects to search for Lo Yu to ask if he would work for the government and help with the administration. Lo Yu declined, saying he had promised to devote his life to researching tea.

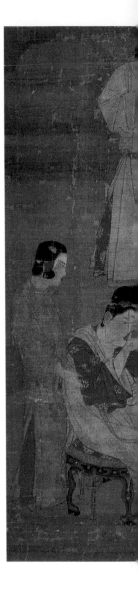

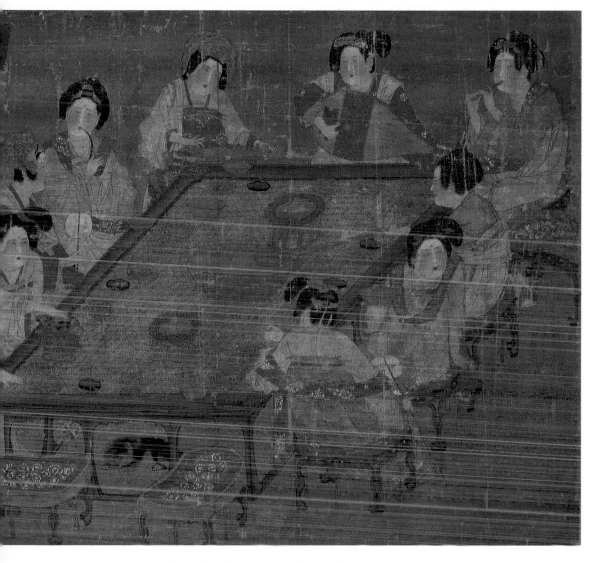

This colorful painting, of elegant Chinese ladies enjoying a feast, music, and a cup of tea, dates from around the 10th century, toward the end of the Tang Dynasty.

The Golden Age of Tea

At this time loose tea leaves were rarely used for making tea as the leaves were steamed and pounded into tea bricks or balls and put into water to brew the tea (see pp. 44–47). Loose leaves were usually given as gifts to kings and important people or presented as rewards to loyal subjects by kings. As the importance of tea grew, the royal houses sent out specialists to search for new varieties of tea plants and develop ways of cultivating them. Others were charged with inventing different ways of preparing and drinking tea. The kings also introduced a tea tax as tea was becoming increasingly popular and more integrated into Chinese manners and customs.

Tea drinking during the Sung Dynasty (A.D. 960–1279) continued the fashion begun in the Tang Dynasty (A.D. 618–907). Emperor Hui Tsung (A.D. 1107–1125) wrote his famous *Ta Kuan Ch'a Lun*, in which he gives accurate details of the skills involved in all aspects of growing, processing, brewing, and drinking tea. Emperor Hui Tsung firmly believed that white tea (see pp. 53–55), although the rarest and hardest to process, was the best tea of all. With the country at peace he encouraged people every-where to enjoy the benefits of tea drinking, as it fostered a lightness of spirit and serenity of mind. Around this time specialists developed ways of preparing loose leaves to make tea — rather than the tea bricks or balls — and people began to brew tea leaves in designated teapots and drink tea from special cups. They discovered that the pottery greatly influenced the taste of the tea and potters began to develop and refine their craftsman-ship. In this way the influence of tea penetrated many aspects of society.

Throughout the Ming Dynasty (1368–1644) research focused on how to preserve tea and simplify preparation methods without compromising its taste. New ways of making strong, heat-resistant, yet fine ceramic teapots were developed. The quality of chinaware was unrivaled and shiploads of porcelain were exported to Europe. Today the Jixing tzu sha tea sets, which contain high iron levels, are still considered the best and are famous worldwide. Around this time tea tasting became a recognized profession and it was fashionable to enter one of the many tea competitions. Awards were presented for the best tea making and tea maker and for the best tea sets. The government also reduced the tea tax and promoted the mass production and cultivation of tea.

During the Ching Dynasty (1644–1911) the spirits of the people in China fell and so too did the popularity of tea. This was due in part to foreign influence, but also to war and the introduction of opium. Not only was very little research carried out on tea but tea-drinking habits changed: whereas tea had always been used to welcome visitors and encourage guests to prolong their stay, now the upper and business classes expected visitors to leave once they had finished their tea.

The Chinese Republic was established in 1911 after the overthrow of the Manchu Dynasty and the People's Republic of China was formed 38 years later in 1949. Over the last 100 years tea has become commercialized and people tend to drink it in combination with other activities. For example, in Fukien teahouses also house the public baths, while in Canton they serve tea with dim sum. Teahouses are also venues for storytelling. Nonetheless, interest in tea for its own sake is rekindling and wealthy people have started to commission research into finding special luxury teas that can be appreciated, as in times past, for their taste alone.

Over many generations tea brewing has become a deep and demanding art, enjoying great periods of renaissance as well as periods of decline. However, tea culture is still very much alive in China and has spread far and wide across the globe (see pp. 24–37). Tea wisdom and customs built up through the ages have been handed down from generation to generation and vary across the different regions in China. Different varieties of tea are grown in different regions and different people have developed their own ways of preparing, serving, and drinking tea. For example, the people south of Xinjiang (Sinkiang) drink tea on its own without adding milk and salt, while people in the north, in Xinjiang, drink tea with milk and salt like the Mongolians. This method is similar to the way English tea is drunk. In southern China people may also add pepper and kuei pi (cassia bark) to their tea and boil the brew for four minutes before pouring and drinking. This brew is considered very healthy, as the pepper improves your appetite and the kuei pi helps when you are short of breath. For maximum benefit drink this brew at least three times a day with meals. The diversity of tea-drinking customs in China is a true reflection of the different historical and cultural identities of each region and the extent to which tea has penetrated every aspect of Chinese society.

Tea-drinking Customs in China

China has many different tea-drinking customs and traditions, some of which are typical of only certain regions and others that are common across the entire country. Selling tea is listed as one of the 72 occupations and in the past there were shops that sold nothing but tea. The Chinese drink tea in numerous ways. Traditionally, many people suckled their tea, which involved taking a spoon of tea and noisily sucking it. This method allowed them to fully appreciate the taste, although today few people drink their tea in this way as it is considered very rude. It is now more common to take extremely small sips from a very small cup to enjoy the tea's aroma to the fullest. Some people drink their tea and then eat the leaves at the bottom of their cup, while others who want to quench their thirst gulp down their tea in big mouthfuls. Thirsty laborers on building sites often buy "big bowl tea" from local tea sellers, as the traditional teacups are normally too small to quench their thirsts. These larger bowls are about the size of a rice bowl.

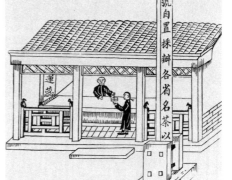

This small French engraving dating from 1928 shows a tea shop in Beijing.

However, drinking tea is not just about appreciating its taste or its ability to refresh the drinker but also an important social event, providing endless opportunities to gossip, discuss business, and perform certain rituals. Whenever people receive guests at their homes they should serve tea as a gesture of welcome, whether or not they know them. If the guest is important, hosts will serve their best quality tea in their best tea set.

In big cities, such as Canton, drinking tea with dim sum has replaced breakfast and is a time for people to socialize and talk business. The word for restaurant in China literally refers to a tea building. The custom of eating snacks with tea has grown out of the villages, where poor people who enjoyed the custom of sharing tea served it with different flour snacks.

Presenting tea gifts is another village custom that spread to the cities. If a young man wanted to court a young woman, his household would send a matchmaker to her house with a gift of tea leaves. The family would make the tea and converse with the matchmaker. If the family drank the tea, this would signal their agreement to the engagement proposal; if they left the tea, this would indicate their refusal. A matchmaker could visit the family three or four times, but if the tea was left untouched on each occasion the young man's household would understand the family's decision. This custom gradually became more elaborate, with matchmakers bringing not only tea but also other "tea gifts," such as wine, livestock, clothes, cakes and biscuits, tea snacks, and even jewelry.

Tea is often drunk as part of special rituals. For example, when a man and a woman marry they share a cup of strong tea. They put a lotus nut and a dried red date in the cup to represent their wish for many children and happiness. Strong tea means their love will also be strong. In the past the wife lived in her husband's family house and served her father- and mother-in-law tea every morning. Today, she serves this "daughter-in-law tea" only on the wedding day.

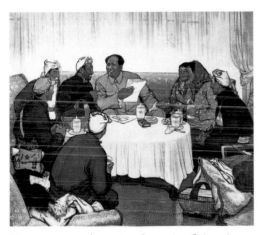

This propaganda poster from the Cultural Revolution is titled "The hearts of Yenan girls turn toward Chairman Mao." It shows the conviviality of the tea table.

There is another tea tradition in China for asking forgiveness of an elder. The person who has made the mistake offers the elder tea and kneels down. The elder shows acceptance of the apology by drinking the tea. To leave the tea is to refuse forgiveness, which is now rare except in very unusual circumstances. A similar ritual is still important for apprenticeships in cookery, carpentry, martial arts, or any other trade, craft, or art. The new pupil kneels down and offers the teacher tea. Drinking the tea is a sign of accepting the student. Similarly, on their first day at school pupils often offer their teacher tea.

On special occasions, such as New Year, the younger generation serve their elders a cup of tea containing a dry red date. This represents prosperity and harmony for the elder. In the south of China this tea is called red date tea, while in the north it is known as yuan pao, or nugget tea.

During the Chinese Revolution when different revolutionary groups wanted to meet in public, they used their tea sets to communicate to which group they belonged. They did this by making coded hand signals when arranging the teacups and pot, and when pouring and drinking the tea.

Today, most Chinese households throughout the world have a small shrine or altar. Every day the family places gifts on the shrine, such as tea, fruit, and incense, in honor of their ancestors or the gods and spirits.

The Spread of Tea from China

Tea reached the height of fashion during the Tang Dynasty and it was around this time that it began to spread outside China, first to Japan and Korea and then to the Middle East. Tea did not reach Europe until the 16th century, about 800 years later, and is often considered the greatest gift that the East has given to the West. Today, in the 21st century, tea is cultivated in a number of different countries throughout the world and exported to many more. Tea is one of the most popular beverages in the world and people all over the world consider it a daily essential.

When China began to export tea the Cantonese word for tea, "ch'a," was often borrowed: the Portuguese who traded in Macao adopted "ch'a," the Russians called it "chai," the Japanese, Hindus, and Persians pronounced it "cha," the Arabs used "shai," and the Turks named it "chay."

Although China has a unified written language, it has always been a large nation with many different dialects. Fukien is a province of Canton and has an international port called X'iamen that exported tea to many parts of Europe. The Fukien dialect word for tea is "te" and it was this pronunciation that the foreign traders used when they took the tea home with them; hence the English word is tea, the Dutch and German use "Tee," the French word is "thé," and the Italians, Spanish, Danish, Norwegians, and Swedes all say "te."

The emergence of tea ceremonies in Japan

At the beginning of the ninth century, Japanese visitors to China took home the fashion of tea. One in particular, the Buddhist monk Dengyo Daishi, studied in China until A.D. 705 and then took back some seeds to his monastery when he returned to Japan. Initially, tea was consumed only by Buddhist monks to keep themselves awake during long periods of meditation, although by the 13th century, tea had grown popular outside the monasteries. The Japanese began their own research on tea and evolved their own tea ceremony, which is very different from the Chinese way of tea. In China, the focus is on enjoying the flavor and taste of the drink itself, whereas in Japan the focus is predominantly on the ceremony.

Zen Buddhism is responsible for the focus of the Japanese way of tea, the "cha do." Cha do places great importance on the harmony of the surroundings, creating an atmosphere of tranquillity and peace, and respecting the tea and the tea set itself – there is a very specific order in

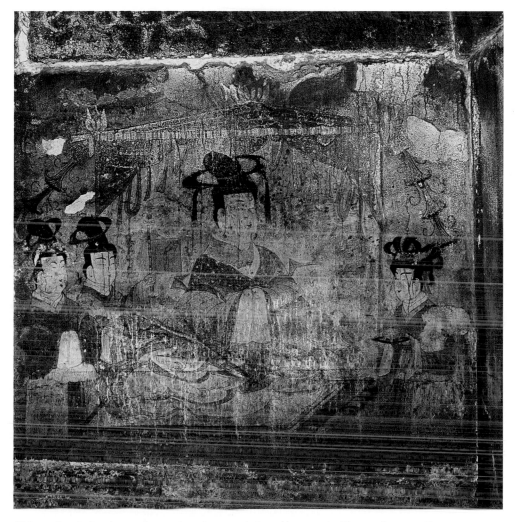

This wall painting in tomb number three at Anhag, Koguryo, in Korea, shows a Korean nobleman being served tea by his wife. It dates from the Three Kingdoms period (A.D. 221–277) when Korea was still part of China.

which to prepare the tea. Cha do is an occasion for teaching manners and protocols, as it shows distinctions between the social classes. In the past a woman had to learn how to perform the tea ceremony before getting married. By the 15th century the aesthetics of drinking tea had been turned into a kind of religion, known as teaism. In *The Book of Tea* published in 1906, Kakuzo Okakura describes teaism as:

"...a cult founded on the adoration of the beautiful among the sordid facts of everyday existence. It inculcates purity and harmony, the mystery of mutual charity, the romanticism of the social order. It is essentially a worship of the imperfect, as it is a tender attempt to accomplish something possible in this impossible thing we know as life."

The tea ceremony involves the host entering the room with the tea set, preparing the tea, and serving it to the guests with some special sweets. The ceremony is artistically entertaining and highly organized. Although it now tends to take place in a designated room in the host's house, in the past the ceremony would be held in a special small outbuilding overlooking the garden. The decor of the room tends to be simple to reflect Zen Buddhism and Zen philosophy, for example a scroll of calligraphy or a drawing might hang on the wall or there might be a vase of carefully arranged flowers. In the middle of the room there is often a small fireplace for making hot water and preparing the tea. The tea itself is made out of green tea powder and hot water; it is usually thin and watery with lots of small bubbles, although it can be very thick.

Korean and Tibetan customs

Around A.D. 820 the people of Ch'a Hsien, now modern Korea, wanted to cultivate their own tea rather than always import it from China. They sent emissaries to China to bring back seeds from tea plants, the skill of growing them, and the technique of preparing tea. Koreans have not evolved their own distinct way of drinking tea but have drawn from the traditions of the Chinese and Japanese.

The Tibetans have a special oily tea called Su Yu Ch'a that they make for very important guests. A Chinese princess from the Tang Dynasty introduced it when she was married into the Tibetan royal family and the recipe was adapted to suit local tastes. To prepare the tea, the host

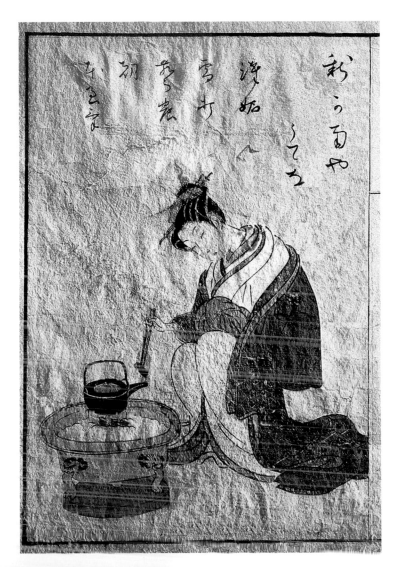

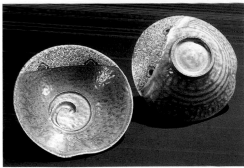

Above This wood block print shows a Japanese lady preparing water for tea.

Left This pair of ceremonial tea bowls date from the Middle Edo period in Japan, which was around the time of the Tang Dynasty (A.D. 618–907).

pounds the leaves and puts them into a long metallic pot to cook for half an hour before adding some yak butter and salt to taste. The pot is then shaken from side to side to make lots of noise and finally poured. The tea is extremely strong and has a very distinctive flavor: you need a strong stomach to drink it.

There is a certain etiquette to drinking Su Yu Ch'a. Once your host has poured you a cup it is considered impolite to drink it all. Instead, you must drink only half the tea and leave the rest unfinished so your host knows you would like some more. If after a few cups you have had enough, you are expected to pour the remainder of your tea onto the floor.

The spread of tea to Mongolia and Russia

During the Tang and Sung Dynasties tea was presented as royal gifts to the Mongolians and in this way became part of their culture. In Mongolia they drink their tea with milk and salt. When the Mongolians expanded into Russia in 1638, they took their tea traditions with them. However, the Mongolians were not the first to bring tea into Russia: in 1618 the Chinese had already given a gift of tea to Tsar Alexis. Thus began a camel caravan trade that covered approximately 11,000 miles — it took almost a year and a half to complete each journey. Tea was extremely popular in Russia and by the end of the 18th century, the Russians were drinking three million pounds of it a year. Because the demand for tea was so high Russia began to cultivate its own tea plantations and by 1900 had stopped importing tea from China. In general, the Russians drink their tea like the Chinese although it can be much stronger. However, they may also add sugar and lemon — some Russians even put the sugar into their mouth before drinking the tea — or else milk, honey, jam, or spices.

Tea traditions in Malaysia and Thailand

In Malaysia and Thailand the people drink their tea the Chinese way although, because of Western influence, they may add milk, sugar, or lemon. The most distinctive feature about Malaysian tea drinking is that their teapots have a very small opening. When they pour tea into a cup they lift the teapot higher and higher to create a long trail of tea, which they call "stretching the tea." The resulting foam and bubbles in the cup introduce more oxygen into the tea and give it a much smoother taste.

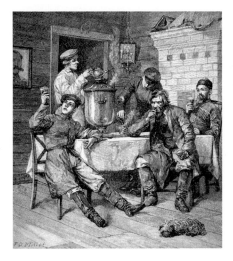

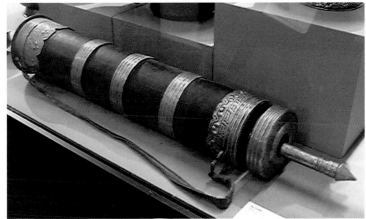

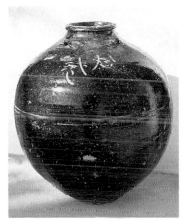

This elaborate wood and brass cylinder is a tea churn from northern India. After boiling the water, tea was poured into it together with butter and sugar. The plunger sticking out of the the cylinder was pushed up and down to mix the brew.

Top This interior of a Russian tea shop dates from around 1007. There is a traditional samovar on the table, a large copper urn with an internal heater.

Above A Sung Dynasty blackware vase with Chinese characters describing the style of tea it contained. Vases like this were taken to Africa from China along the silk routes and by the Arab coastal Indian Ocean trade.

Right These senior lamas are performing a tea ceremony in their yurt, which is attached to a temple in the Mongolian People's Republic.

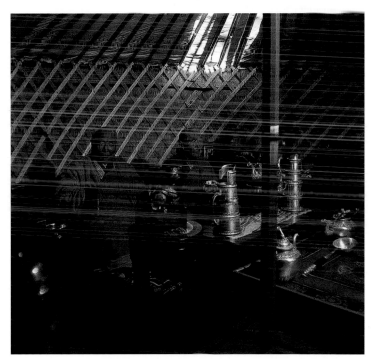

The Indonesian tea market

Although Chinese tea plants are mentioned in Indonesian botanical literature from around the 1820s, the Dutchman J. I. L. L. Jacobson is largely responsible for establishing tea in Indonesia. He recognized the growing popularity of tea in Europe and its market potential. Jacobson visited China several times in order to learn the art of cultivating tea, then between 1827 and 1833 he brought a great number of professional Chinese tea farmers to Indonesia, as well as many tea sets and tea instruments. He established large tea plantations and began to mass-produce tea for export to Europe. The tea plant he brought to Indonesia was the variety from the Mo Yi mountain. Because of his expansion of the tea market in Indonesia, the Indonesians call Jacobson "the father of Indonesian tea."

Tea exploits in India and Sri Lanka

The tea brought from China to India and Sri Lanka was a red tea. Planted in the local soil the tea tasted completely different and much stronger than the original imported tea. Because of their preference for sweet things, locals added milk and sugar as well as other ingredients, such as ginger, mint, and tou k'ou (nutmeg). Sometimes the tea is cooked instead of simply infused in water, which helps to bring out the flavor of the tea.

By the late 17th century the people of India had become experts at growing very beautiful tea plants, but had no knowledge of how to prepare the leaves. In 1728 Holland's East India Company recognized this talent and decided to mass-produce Chinese tea in India and Ceylon, now Sri Lanka. They hired a large number of Chinese tea makers, imported the plants, and set about preparing the tea leaves the Chinese way.

In 1833 the British East India Company lost its monopoly over the tea trade with China and began to establish tea plantations in Assam in northern India. At first the British planters imported Chinese seed and Chinese experts showed them how to cultivate the tea plants and process the leaves. However, soon they began to mass-produce the Assam variety that Major Robert Bruce and his brother Charles had discovered growing indigenously in 1823. The Assam variety was much taller with heavier leaves and more suited to the Indian climate and soil conditions. In 1839 Assam tea went on sale in London for the first time.

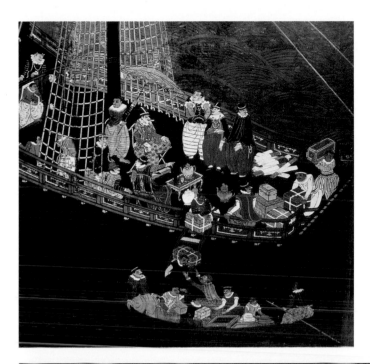

Left This detail from a Japanese folding screen shows a harbor scene with Portuguese tea merchants arriving in Japan. The Indian servants unload the boat while the merchant sits drinking tea on deck. Edo Period, early 17th century.

Below This Chinese painting shows a tea auction in a Hong Kong warehouse circa 1800. The European merchants are negotiating tea prices.

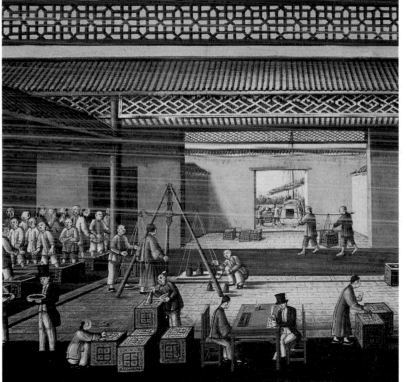

The British went on to introduce a management system to optimize tea production, as well as machinery, including rollers, firers, and dryers. Tea making became more efficient and the process was simplified. As Edward Money wrote in his "Essay on the Cultivation and Manufacture of Tea" in 1872:

"Fortunately for the tea enterprise, the more manufacture is studied, the more does it appear that to make good tea is a very simple process."

The British initiative made India the largest producer and exporter of tea, pushing it ahead of China, which is now the second largest.

Tea fashion in Europe

No one is entirely sure whether Portugal or Holland was the first country to bring tea to Europe. At the beginning of the 17th century the Portuguese imported Chinese tea to Lisbon, which they sold on to France and Holland. Meanwhile, the Dutch also imported Japanese tea via their colony on Java in the Dutch East Indies, which they too sold on, not only to France but also to Germany. The Dutch were great tea enthusiasts and by the middle of the 17th century it was already common to drink afternoon tea.

Rumors of tea and its benefits had been reaching England from the Continent for a few years before Thomas Garraway's announcement on September 9, 1658 of a tea auction in London. In the same edition of the London newspaper that also broke the news of Cromwell's death he writes:

"That excellent and by all Physicians approved drink called by the Chineans Tcha, by other nations Tay alias Tea, is sold at the Sultaness Head, a cophee house in Sweeting's Rents by the Royal Exchange, London."

The British enthusiastically adopted the Dutch habit of drinking afternoon tea and it was not long before the tea fashion took over London's coffeehouses: everybody who could drank tea. Samuel Pepys was partial to tea as was Catherine of Braganza of Portugal, who married King Charles II of England in 1661. She served her friends afternoon tea and very soon tea became the talk of aristocratic drawing rooms across the capital. However, it was the Duchess of Bedford who left the most pro-found mark on English tea-drinking habits: she could not abide the long interval between the midday and evening meal, so she introduced the custom of eating cakes with afternoon tea.

The ever-increasing demand for tea and the promise of high profit mar-gins meant it would be more economical for the English to trade directly with China rather than import tea from Holland. The British East India Company, which had been founded by royal charter in 1600, sent a few shipments of goods to Canton in China to trade for tea, and thus began the successes of one of the most powerful companies the world has seen: under its influence British India was established, Hong Kong and Singapore were founded, and the fortunes of Elihu Yale were forged (Elihu Yale sub-sequently founded Yale University). The British East India flag is also said to be the inspiration for America's Stars and Stripes.

In 1664, the British East India Company brought from China 2 lb 2 oz (964 g) of super grade A Chinese tea leaves, which it presented as gifts to the British monarchy. In 1666, it asked a Dutchman to deliver 22 lb 12 oz (10.3 kg) of special Chinese tea leaves to the British royal family to thank them for allowing them to trade — the monarchy had given them control over the entire English tea market. In 1715 the British East India Company purchased a large amount of lower grade green tea from China and sold it directly to the public, not through coffeehouses, but via special tea stores. In later years world-famous stores, including Harrods and Fortnum and Mason, would start out in business as tea and grocery stores.

Britain and the American tea trade

In 1690 Boston became the first place to sell tea in America. Only red tea and Wu I tea were sold and it was another 20 years before green tea and other teas went on sale. Until 1770 tea was mainly smuggled in by Dutch traders, as the British levied high import duties on all products in their American colonies. Although many import duties were lifted in 1770 tea continued to be taxed. Around this time the British East India Company was experiencing financial problems. In order to strengthen its monopoly Lord North passed the Tea Act in 1773 to make English tea more mar-ketable in America. The Tea Act was drawn up in such a way that the British

This engraving dated 1790 is taken from a painting by Morland. It depicts a wealthy English family taking tea in one of the popular public tea gardens. These were fashionable in London and other large European cities at this time. The whole family enjoys the occasion and even the dog is offered a sandwich.

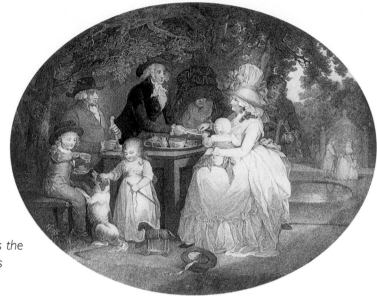

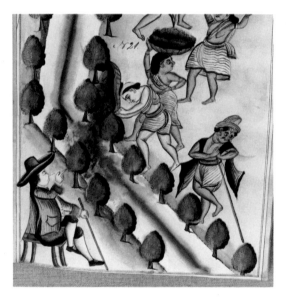

Above This late 18th-century Indian painting shows an early tea planation in Imperial India. An English gentleman planter sits smoking as he watches a group of bare-breasted women pick tea leaves. This plantation may have belonged to the British East India Company.

Right By the late 19th century, under British Imperial rule, there were many tea plantations in the north Indian territories of Assam and Darjeeling. Tea production had become a highly organized and partially mechanized process to meet the rising demands of the home market for cheap tea. This engraving was published in the March 1876 edition of the popular Illustrated London News magazine. It shows the various stages of tea cultivation and production in India at that time.

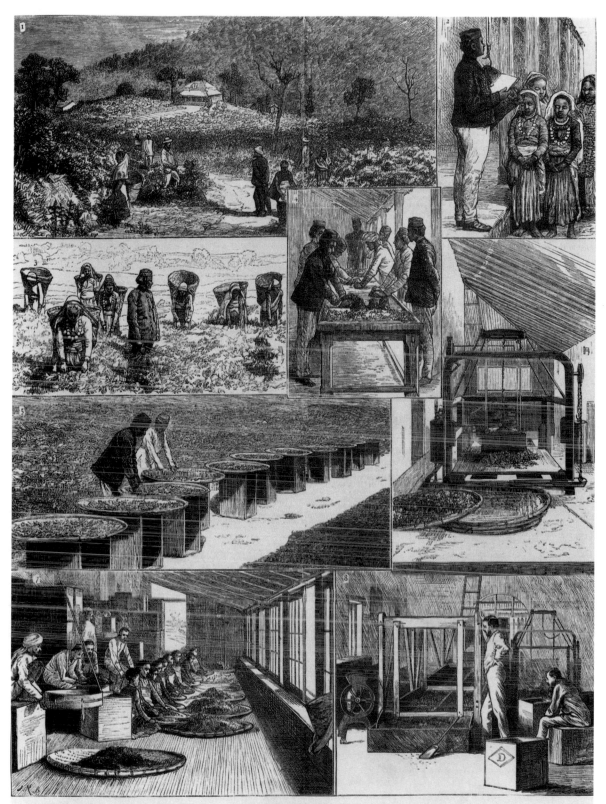

1. Ging Tea Plantation, Darjeeling.—2. Weighing the Leaf.—3. Plucking the Leaf.—4. Rolling by Hand.—5. Withering in the Sun.—6. Rolling by Machinery.—7. Withering in the Factory.—8. Sorting by Machinery.

TEA CULTIVATION IN BRITISH INDIA

> **BOSTON**, *December* 2, 1773.
>
> WHEREAS it has been reported that a Permit will be given by the Custom-House for Landing the Tea now on Board a Vessel laying in this Harbour, commanded by Capt. HALL: THIS is to Remind the Publick, That it was solemnly voted by the Body of the People of this and the neighbouring Towns assembled at the Old-South Meeting House on Tuesday the 30th Day of *November*, that the said Tea never should be landed in this Province, or pay one Farthing of Duty: And as the aiding or assisting in procuring or granting any such Permit for landing the said Tea or any other Tea so circumstanced, or in offering any Permit when obtained to the Master or Commander of the said Ship, or any other Ship in the same Situation, must betray an inhuman Thirst for Blood, and will also in a great Measure accelerate Confusion and Civil War: This is to assure such public Enemies of this Country, that they will be considered and treated as Wretches unworthy to live, and will be made the first Victims of our just Resentment.
>
> *The* PEOPLE.
>
> N. B. Captain *Bruce* is arrived laden with the same detestable Commodity: and 'tis peremptorily demanded of him, and all concerned, that they comply with the same Requisitions.

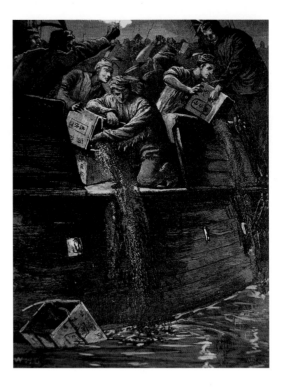

Above American patriots published this notice on December 2, 1773. It warns against the landing of British ships carrying tea in Boston Harbor.

Right On December 16 the patriots took direct action, tipping the tea into the harbor.

East India Company paid the duties but could still sell tea at a much lower price than all its rivals. The British East India Company tea shipments and British taxation laws became symbols of British tyranny to the Americans. Resentment grew and came to a head on the night of the Boston Tea Party.

The Boston Tea Party

On the night of December 16, 1773, the same year that the Tea Act was introduced, a large number of people dressed as Native Americans climbed aboard a ship owned by the British East India Company and threw all the tea overboard into the sea. This was repeated the following spring in New York, in April 1774. In response to this uprising the British Parliament introduced four acts to punish the Americans, known collectively as the Intolerable Acts. One of them, the Boston Port Deal, shut off the sea trade in Boston in order to pay for the destroyed tea. This was one of the catalysts of the American War of Independence in 1775.

In 1784, the Americans built their first ship for trading with China. They sailed to Canton and brought back tea, silk, and chinaware. The mission was so successful and so profitable that the man in charge became an

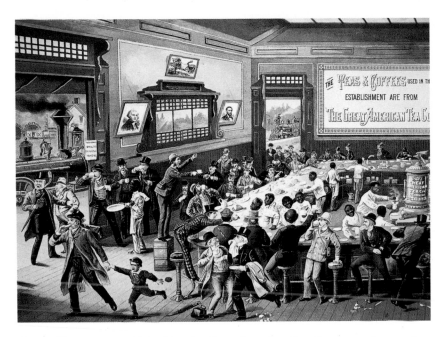

Above This poster published by the Great American Tea Company shows rail passengers hurrying to drink cups of tea at an early fast food counter.

ambassador in the American embassy in China. This was the first foreign embassy in Canton. From this time onward America sent shipments to and from China. This contributed to the growth and prosperity of the shipping industry in America. In 1815 the first tea clipper sailed from New York, returning less than eight months later and in so doing almost halved the time taken by the ships of the British East India Company. The British countered with their first clipper, the *Stornoway*, which managed to carry as much as 1,000,000 lb (454,000 kg) of tea and to cut the journey time from China to less than 100 days.

Despite several unsuccessful attempts to import seed and cultivate tea at home, America continues to drink tea in large quantities: it is the world's second largest importer of tea, although coffee remains the country's most common drink. Americans are particularly partial to iced tea, which was invented by Englishman Richard Blechynden at the St. Louis Worlds Fair in 1904. Failing utterly in his attempts to sell hot tea because of a heat wave, in desperation he poured hot tea into a glass with ice cubes. It was an instant hit and spread in popularity across America. Later, honey and sugar were added for extra flavoring, with some people even adding a dash of alcohol to improve the taste.

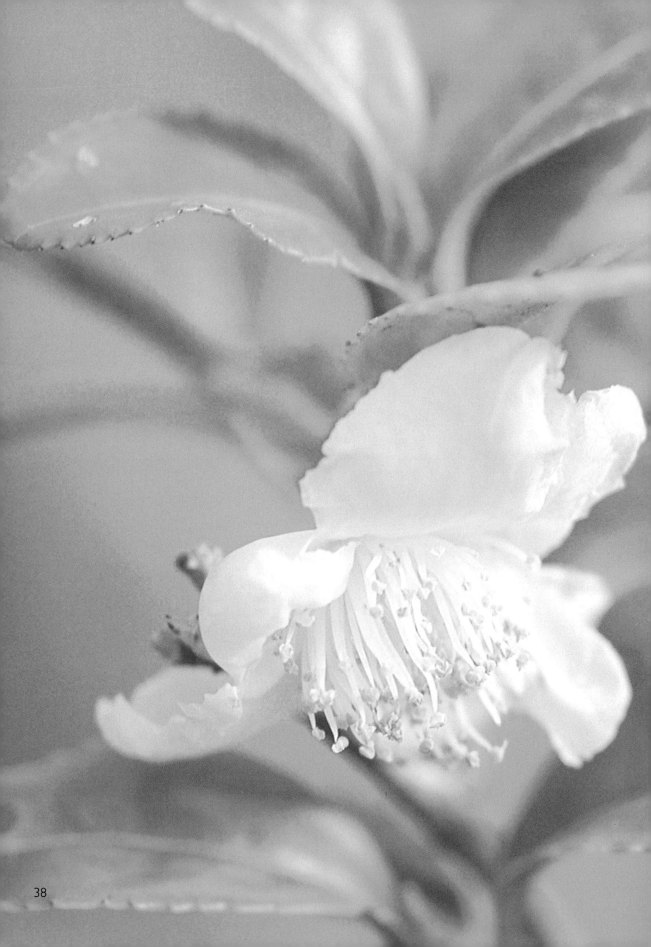

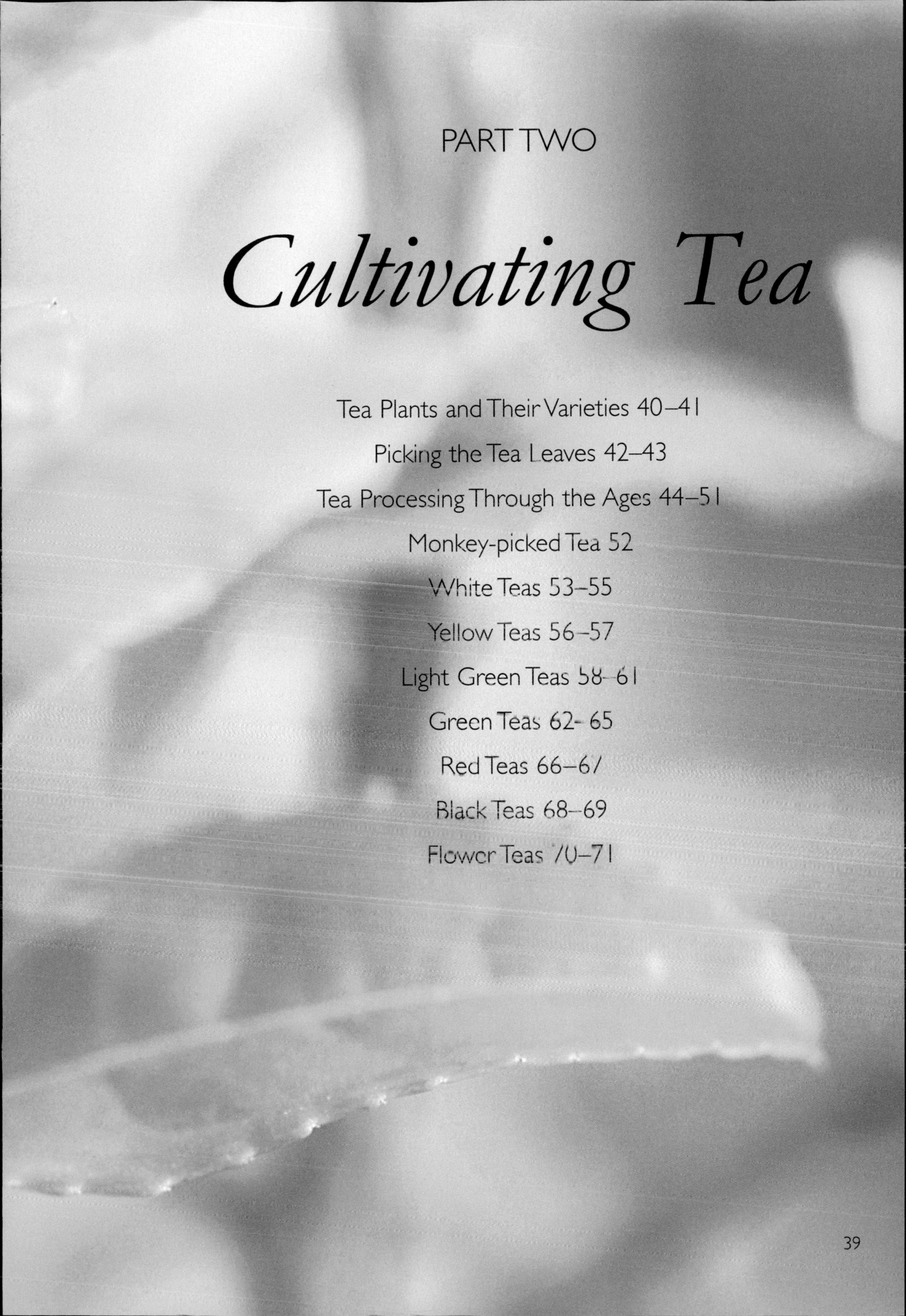

PART TWO

Cultivating Tea

Tea Plants and Their Varieties 40–41

Picking the Tea Leaves 42–43

Tea Processing Through the Ages 44–51

Monkey-picked Tea 52

White Teas 53–55

Yellow Teas 56–57

Light Green Teas 58–61

Green Teas 62–65

Red Teas 66–67

Black Teas 68–69

Flower Teas 70–71

Tea Plants and Their Varieties

Tea plants are either wild or cultivated and in China are subdivided into six different types: white, yellow, light green, green, red, and black. In the West, green tea and light green tea are not distinguished: both are classified as green tea. Although this chapter offers general guidelines for the coloring, aroma, and taste of the six types, you will often find that the tea you choose to drink looks, smells, and tastes quite different. This is because within the six types of tea there are many different varieties and grades.

A common misunderstanding is to equate fermented tea with black tea, unfermented with green tea, and semi-fermented with Oolong tea. Chinese tea culture does not categorize tea in this way, rather in terms of the kind of tea leaf and the way in which the tea is prepared. To truly understand a pinch of tea you have to know its type and variety, how it started out in seed, how it was cultivated and picked, how the leaves were separated, and how they were cooked and packaged.

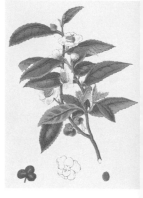

The Chinese camellia

The Latin name for tea, *Camellia sinensis*, literally means Chinese camellia. A camellia is an ornamental Asian shrub with rose-like flowers. Like the ornamental camellia, tea plants are evergreens. Their leaves vary in shape and size: some are as large as hands while others are as small as needles. There are three kinds of tea plants, namely China, Assam, and Cambodia. The Cambodia plant is a single-stemmed tree that has been naturally interbred with other varieties. It can grow as tall as 16 feet (5 meters). The Assam trees are also single stemmed and grow between 20 and 60 feet (6 and 18 meters) high depending on the sub-variety. If regularly cut or plucked, its economic lifespan is about 40 years. The Chinese variety has multi-stemmed bushes and if left can grow as high as 9 feet (2.75 meters). However, it is only allowed to grow to half this height. This variety can withstand cold winters and produce good quality tea for at least 100 years.

Like any other plant the tea plant has roots, stem, leaves, flowers, and fruit, and is dependent on sunlight, air, water, and soil. However, where a tea plant is cultivated is also important, as the same type of plant growing in different places produces different teas. This is because the tea plant adjusts itself to the local soil and climate, which in turn affects the flavor. China has several hundred types of tea plant although only a hundred of these are regularly drunk — no other country has as many.

Sunshine, fertile soil, and a hot climate are not always the key to successful tea plants. Some, such as the cold summit Oolong tea (p. 60) and the large white tea in Fukien, prefer a cold, frozen climate, while others need only a little water or less fertile soil. There are also mountain teas that thrive at high altitudes and rocky teas that prefer the cracks of rocks and cliff faces. Tea plants should be not be grown too close together as they get in each other's way and fight for light and soil. Every year tea farmers cut the plants three times to remove branches and force the plant to grow horizontally. This encourages more branches and more leaves and allows the farmer to pick the plants more easily. However, it takes three years before you can start plucking a baby plant.

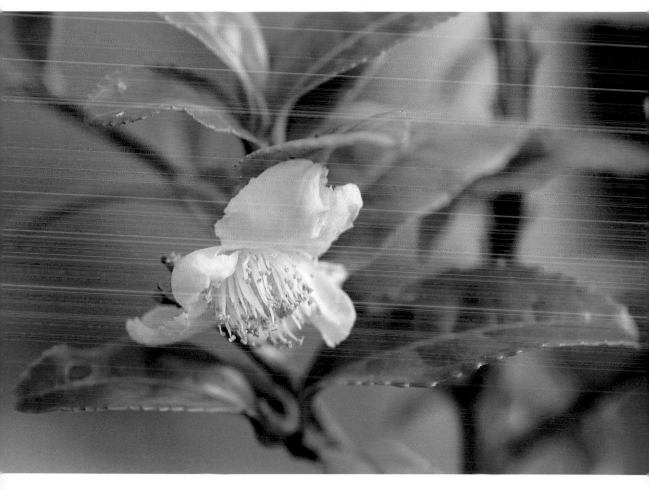

Picking the Tea Leaves

At harvest time in China, the leaves are plucked by hand, as there are different quality leaves on every single plant. Other countries do use machinery, but because machines cannot identify and separate the different leaves machine-picked tea can only produce a tea of average quality. Hand-picking is a very delicate and tedious process. It was started by traditional Chinese doctors who collected wild herbs in the mountains. Eventually, as the demand for tea grew and plantations were established, more people were needed. Because men tend to have clumsy fingers, large numbers of young girls were and still are trained to pluck the leaves.

In China some teas are extremely expensive while others are relatively inexpensive, even for the same kind of tea. The quality and price of the leaves are also dependent on the time of day that the tea is picked. In general, the tea leaves are plucked two or three times a day. The best quality leaves are picked at the first light of dawn until 7 A.M., before the sun fully rises between 7 and 8 or even 9 A.M., and again at sunset when the sun's heat is not very strong. However, some farmers dislike the early morning mist because the moisture makes the drying process more difficult so they pluck at midday when the sun is much stronger. These teas are cruder and of lower quality. The seasons also affect tea quality: spring produces the best leaves and as the months progress between spring and summer the quality falls. Traditionally, no one plucks tea in autumn and winter so the plants can rejuvenate themselves, although today they pluck the leaves in all four seasons to maintain year-round production.

When harvesting the leaves the picker uses the middle finger and thumb, known as the orchard hand sign, to lightly hold the leaves and pluck them from the plant in a steady movement. This keeps damage to the leaves at a minimum. The best tea leaves are the smallest, most delicate ones at the tip of each shoot. Shaped like the head of a very small spear, these leaves make very expensive teas — in the past only kings could afford them. This is why they are called offering teas. All the other leaves on the plant are called flags and the quality of leaves is judged by the flags from which they are picked. The few leaves from the spear produce supergrade tea. The next best quality teas are those using the spear and the first flag leaves, then the spear and the first two flags. The higher the flag number the lower the tea quality. Leaves used for green tea are usually from the spear and first few flags of the tea plant, whereas black teas often use them from third, fourth, or higher flags.

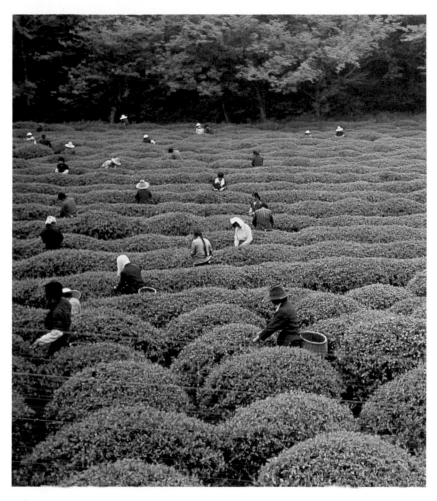

Women picking tea in Hangzhou, Zhejiang province, China. The finest teas are said to be those picked by young girls before sunrise.

Tea farmers always monitor the growth of the tea leaves. Too much growth reduces the quality and the grade and so they have to sell it more cheaply. They also have to be vigilant for harmful insects that could ruin the entire plantation: there are over 150 different species of insects and over 380 kinds of fungi that can attack tea plants. If farmers find an infestation they cannot use any pesticides; the most they can do is break off the infected branch or use smoke to get rid of the insects. Pesticides ruin the taste and flavor of the infected plant and those surrounding it: the farmers would rather burn the tea plant and start again.

When the tea leaves are plucked they have to be immediately processed and prepared, as any delay affects the quality and the price of the tea drops. Traditionally, tea farmers work intensively for half a year during spring and summer and rest and relax for the second half of the year.

Tea Processing Through the Ages

The first proper processing system was developed during the Tang Dynasty (A.D. 618–907). At this time the tea plants grew only in the wild and their leaves were collected by doctors who went to the mountains looking for herbs. After separating the good leaves from the bad, they were prepared for drinking. This process involved several stages.

The first was called Steaming the Tea, when a big, porous bamboo tray was placed above a wok of hot water and the raw tea leaves were spread thinly over it and steamed.

The second stage was called Grinding the Tea. While they were still hot from the steaming process, the tea leaves were ground in a special basin and smashed into a pulp called tea mud. The tea mud was poured onto a cloth, which was then placed into a circular, square, or more artistically shaped mold. The mold was usually made of metal, although some were made of wood.

The third stage was called Smacking the Tea. The metallic or wooden tea mold was fixed into a larger mold made of rock and a flat metallic object was used to smack the top of the tea mud. This compressed the tea and made it thinner. Next, the cloth containing the now hardening tea mud was lifted out of the mold and the mud was returned to the bamboo tray. This was placed in the open air to dry in the sun. When it had dried, the hard tea mud was called a group tea and was ready for consumption. Group teas shaped in blocks were called tea bricks, while circular or disc-shaped group teas were known as tea cakes.

Although group teas were dried in the sun they still contained moisture and had to be baked to prevent them from rotting. A hole was drilled in the group tea, a bamboo rod pulled through it, and it was placed in a hot oven. Traditionally, the oven was a 2-foot- (60-cm-) deep underground ditch. The tea groups were strung together like beans and distinguished by different weights of string known as the upper string, medium string, and small string. The upper string was heavier duty and held the largest tea bricks or discs and the smallest held the lightest. The largest tea groups were used for exporting and long-distance trading.

The final stage was designed to prevent the flavor from deteriorating. The tea was placed in a bamboo basket with papers glued around the outside. On damp days a container of hot burned ash was placed in the middle of the basket to prevent moisture from entering the tea.

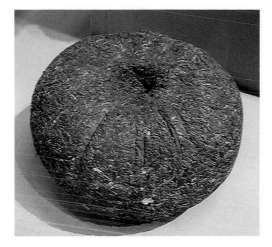

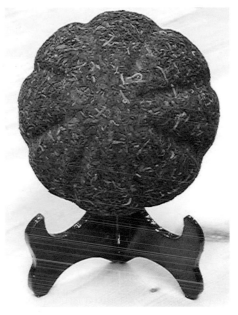

These Polee tea balls (see also p. 64) can be preserved for up to 40 years. Polee tea is extremely popular in Canton and in spite of its brown appearance is a green tea. To use the tea you break off a small piece with a hammer, which you then gently tap to loosen the leaves. Tea bricks or balls are stored either by wrapping them in paper or simply leaving them as they are. However, they must be kept in a well-aired, dry, dark place.

The Golden Age of Tea (A.D. 960–1279)

The Sung emperors were great tea enthusiasts and sent out specialists to study tea cultivation and to refine the tea-making process. One emperor was so partial to tea that he wrote a book on the subject and hired many people to find new kinds of tea plant. Under the Sung Dynasty professionals developed over 100 different kinds of tea and tea fashion reached a new peak. The quality of tea dramatically increased and the tea-making process became more skill-oriented and labor-intensive and therefore more expensive. By the end of the dynasty, the Chinese had discovered how to make tea with loose tea leaves, which is how we still make tea today, although making tea with tea balls and bricks remained popular.

Making tea bricks and balls in the Sung Dynasty

Young girls and women were trained to pick the tea leaves from cultivated tea plants using the orchard hand sign (see p. 42). Specialists also discovered that the time of day they picked the leaves was important: tea picked early in the morning before the sun had fully risen and when the moisture of the morning mist was nurturing the leaves had a better fragrance and color, and made a clearer brew.

When the tea had been picked, a second group of specially trained people floated the leaves on water in order to separate the shoots according to size: the smaller ones were of higher quality and value than the larger ones. The fact that the leaves of a single spear were further divided into five grades shows just how sensitive and knowledgeable the Sung Dynasty Chinese were in their appreciation of tea. After separating the leaves they were steamed. Controlling the temperature of the fire was very important for if the fire was too strong and the heat too high then the leaves would turn an off-yellow color and the resulting tea would be very mild and tasteless. Conversely, if the heat was too low, the tea would have a raw, grassy, unpleasant smell. The steamed tea leaves are known as "Ch'a Huang," which literally means yellow tea.

The next stage was known as Squeezing the Tea. Cold water was poured over the steamed leaves several times to cool them down. Once cool, the leaves were put into a cloth and placed in a small compressor to squeeze out the water. Next the leaves were placed into a larger, more powerful compressor to squeeze out an oily and viscous fluid. The cloth full of leaves was repeatedly removed, hand pressed, rolled, and returned to the compressor until no more fluid appeared. The tea leaves processed in this way had a stronger, better preserved taste.

The fifth stage was called Grinding the Tea. The tea leaves were poured into a large earthen basin that had many small ridges inside it. Strong men with powerful wrists then ground the tea in the basin with long hardwood stumps. They had to add water to the tea powder and different kinds of tea needed different amounts of water. The smaller and more evenly the leaves were broken down the better quality it became. These tea powders were used as a spice to flavor cooking dishes such as soups or, after adding hot water, as an instant tea. The wet tea powders were then poured into molds to form tea bricks, tea cakes, or tea balls.

The last stage was called "Kou Huang," literally passing yellow. The molded tea was placed in the oven and baked at a high temperature. When it was hot enough it was immediately dipped into a pot of hot water and baked again. This was repeated three times. Finally, the tea was baked one last time over a gentle heat, dipped into boiling water, and placed in a sealed room. Here, the tea was fanned to keep the room at a constant temperature and humidity. This process made the tea appear more silky.

Loose-leaf tea

By the Yüan Dynasty (1279–1368) tea bricks and tea balls were no longer popular in China. Instead of steaming the leaves to get rid of the raw, grassy smell from the tea leaves, they stir-fried them in a hot wok. By the Ching Dynasty (1644–1911) nobody made tea bricks or tea balls and only a minority made small tea cakes. Everyone else made only the loose tea that we drink today. Today, tea makers still use the stir-frying method. Stir-frying the leaves is only a part of what is an extremely complicated process and requires great skill. Depending on the variety, the leaves are processed to be unfermented, semi-fermented, or fermented. The method modern Chinese tea makers use today is similar to the method that was already in use by the Ching Dynasty.

Making semi-fermented tea is the most complicated of the three processes. After plucking, the leaves are spread thinly on a large surface under a hot sun or are blown by hot air so that all the moisture in them quickly evaporates. For this to happen, the temperature must remain constant at around 86 °F (30 °C). It usually takes between 10 and 30 minutes. To dry the leaves evenly, the tea makers regularly turn them until they lose their shiny appearance, begin to curl up, and release a particular fragrance. The leaves are then taken indoors for further fermentation.

The tea leaves are left alone indoors for an hour and then the tea maker gently mixes the leaves with his hands and uses his senses to judge the quality. He feels the texture, moisture, and softness of the leaves. He sniffs the leaves for any raw, grassy smell and watches for any yellowing, which is a bad sign. This period of fermentation also involves another stage, known as Swinging Green. When the tea maker mixes the leaves they rub against each other, which makes the leaf cells break down and allows more oxygen to enter. The way and the extent to which the leaves are rubbed against each other requires great skill, as it has a direct

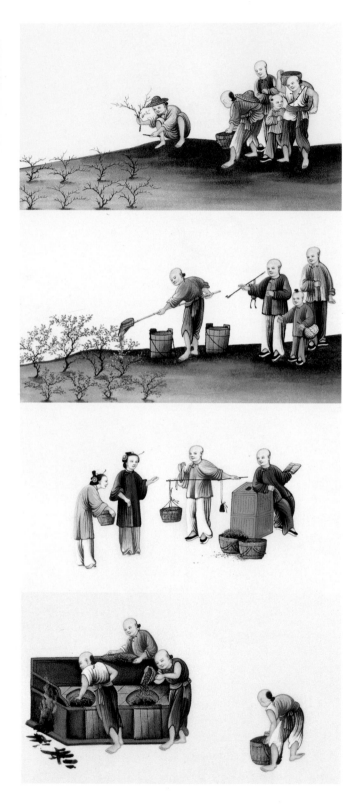

These 19th-century silk paintings are part of a series of 12 paintings that illustrate the traditional way of cultivating and preparing tea.

The first painting, top left, shows workers carefully planting stem cuttings of tea plants at regular intervals.

In the second picture, the workers are mulching the healthy young bushes with composted material.

The third picture shows two women pickers having their leaves weighed; presumably their wages were determined by the weight of the tea they picked.

The fourth picture illustrates the Stir-frying Green stage of tea processing, which stops the fermentation process. The tea makers vary the heat of the wok, their stir-frying technique, and the cooking time according to the variety of tea. Highly skilled tea makers can judge the progress of the tea leaves with their sensitive fingertips.

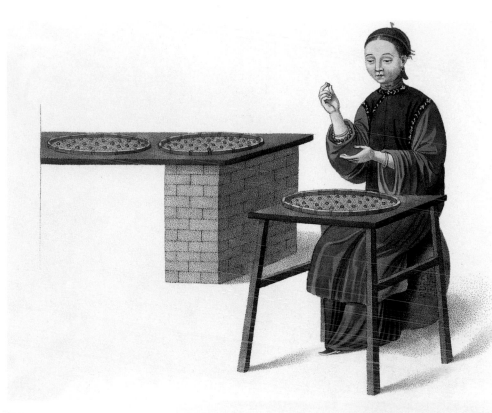

Above This large engraving appears in an English book (circa 1800) called The Costume of China. *The elegantly dressed Chinese woman is hand rolling tea leaves into special little balls, known as dragon balls.*

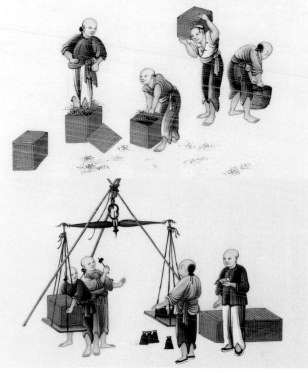

Top right The fifth silk painting in this series shows tea leaves being carefully stored in wooden crates for transportation.

Bottom right In the final painting shown here workers are weighing the boxes of tea on a traditional fulcrum scale. The tea will then be sold.

influence on the final flavor and taste of the tea leaves. Every hour, the tea maker returns to mix and check the tea leaves. The number of times he has to do this depends on the type of tea, the progress of the leaves — the leaves get rougher and stronger throughout the process — and the tea maker's spirit and judgment. If he mixes them too vigorously or his mixing technique is crude, the leaves will be damaged: they will retain water, look dusty, taste bitter, and therefore make very low-quality tea. Equally, if the leaves are not mixed enough, the distinct taste of the semi-fermented leaves will be lost and replaced by a raw, grassy taste.

Stir-frying the loose leaves

The next stage in traditional processing is called Stir-frying Green, when the leaves are literally stir-fried in a large wok. This process stops the leaves from further fermentation, gets rid of any moisture or lingering raw, grassy smell, and seals in the distinct semi-fermented flavor. In Stir-frying Green, the wok has to be kept at a very high temperature. In order to make a good tea, the fire underneath the wok is carefully controlled so the wok is evenly heated. While inexperienced tea makers always burn their hands during this stage, more experienced ones can continously mix leaves with their hands, feeling the texture, smelling the aromas released, and monitoring the color of the tea. The skill involved is extraordinary: different kinds of leaves have to be stir-fried at different temperatures and the technique and number of times they are stir-fried also varies. It is hardly surprising that traditional tea makers, particularly in the past, were highly regarded.

The right amount of cooking, or stir-frying, seals the aroma in the leaves for a long time and means that when the leaves are brewed in water they will produce a good color. If they are undercooked, the leaves will quickly lose their aroma when stored and be left with a raw, grassy smell; if they are overcooked, the tea leaves will feel spiky, sharp, and have a burned smell. An expert tea maker can stir-fry the tea so that the aroma produced is comparable to the fragrance of flowers — it is said that the aroma can even attract bees. Nowadays people tend to blend flavors into tea to create aroma but these are not comparable to the natural aroma of a good tea produced by a skilled tea maker.

Killing Green is a modernized version of stir-frying that uses machinery. Although the machines used for this stage can set the right temperature and the cooking time, they cannot feel and control the texture of the leaves or judge them by their aroma. For this reason, the Killing Green process can only produce common teas. The stir-frying process is still used for the good quality and supergrade teas.

At the end of the Stir-frying or Killing Green stage the tea leaves are curled from the heat, although they are still recognizable as individual leaves. The next stage shapes them together to make them easier to store. If the leaves are not shaped they will soon break down into smaller pieces and become valueless tea dust. This stage also removes the last remaining moisture from the leaves so that the tea leaves quickly release their flavor when brewed.

Shaping the leaves

As soon as the tea maker has finished stir-frying the leaves or the machines have completed the Killing Green process, the leaves are removed and immediately shaped. Traditionally this was all done by hand, but even today there are some teas that cannot be shaped by machines. When shaping the leaves by hand, the tea maker wraps the leaves in a towel, which he rolls up and presses in a particular way, depending on the shape required. Normally the leaves are pressed into balls or sticks.

Once the leaves have been shaped, the tea maker spreads them thinly over a surface to loosen them and prevent them from becoming clustered into one big ball. Although shaping the tea in this way helps preserve the leaves, it is also important for the aesthetic appreciation of the tea, an important part of the tea ceremony.

In the final stage, the shaped leaves are placed in a very hot oven and baked. They are then taken out, spread onto a surface and allowed to cool before being returned to the oven. This ensures that the leaves are baked evenly and prevents further fermentation. (Further fermentation would affect the flavor and quality of the leaves.) Baking the leaves twice also reduces the amount of moisture in the leaves: by the time the leaves have been fully processed the water content is three percent of what it was when they were first picked. In its final form the tea is dry and light in weight. It can be stored and preserved for a long time without losing its flavor. The whole process, from the plucking of the leaves to the final cooking, is continuous and the tea makers have to work day and night, nonstop, to ensure that the leaves make the finest quality tea for tea drinkers to enjoy all over the world.

Monkey-picked Tea

Monkey-picked tea leaves are famous and get their name from the fact that trained monkeys have to pick them — the name does not refer to a particular type of tea. In general, monkey-picked teas are wild tea plants that grow in inaccessible places, such as on high cliff faces, and to harvest them people train special monkeys.

The most famous monkey-picked tea is Yang Hsien Yün Wu, and even Lo Yu (see pp. 16–18), the patron of tea, declared it the world's number one tea. The history of Yang Hsien Yün Wu tea also reveals how monkeys came to be used to pick and collect wild teas.

There was a poor tea maker named Yang Hsien, who lived in Jixing, the same place that produces the famous purple sand tea sets (see p. 81). To earn a living, he used to pluck and prepare tea leaves for rich people. One day in the mountains he found an abandoned baby monkey, so he brought it home and looked after it. They soon became attached to each other and wherever he went the monkey went too.

Some time later, when he was hunting in the mountains, he noticed a tea plant growing high up on a cliff and shrouded in clouds and mist. He tried to climb up to pick the leaves of this tea plant, but it was too difficult and he gave up. On seeing this, the monkey climbed up and collected the leaves from the plant, imitating the poor tea maker's action. When the man returned home he made the tea and it tasted good. The tea was named after him and the cloud and mist (Yün Wu) where he saw the tea plant growing.

White Teas

White teas are slightly fermented and there are only a handful of different varieties. The leaves are paler than other teas and the brewed tea is also paler in color. Some plants appear to have white, hairy fur on their leaves, while others look as though they are covered with ash. Shou Mei, Pai Hao Yin Chin, and Pai Mu Tan are the most popular and best known kinds of white teas.

The fragrance of white teas is much weaker than that of other teas and in order to enjoy it, people usually hold the cup in their hands and bring it close to their mouth before they drink. Instead of having a solid, dominant aroma like other types of tea, white teas tend to have a much more subtle, lingering fragrance: it is like in autumn when you take a deep breath and you can still sense a touch of summer in the air; or when you play a musical instrument, suddenly stop, and for a long moment feel the music continuing, as if it were haunting the space.

Similarly, a white tea brew does not have a distinct color tone, although it may have a touch of yellow, green, or red. When you drink white tea it seems quite tasteless — as if you were drinking hot water with a slightly milder and more subtle taste than normal. However, after a while you will become aware of a subtle change in your breath and at the back of your mouth. You will taste a soft, nourishing sweetness and eventually experience a similar sensation down your throat. Afterward, try taking a sip of hot water and you will notice that white tea is not tasteless but is actually quite sweet with its own individual flavor.

What white tea offers is a bittersweet aftertaste that persists on your tongue, throat, and mouth. In Chinese this is called "fragrance preserved between your teeth." Because white tea is so weak in aroma and taste it is not very popular, although better known than yellow tea (see pp. 56–57).

There is a fairy tale about a white tea called Pai Hao Yin Chin. In Fujian in China there was once a drought and nothing grew for many seasons. A plague started in the villages and settlements and lots of people died.

As the situation got worse the elders told the story of a holy plant that grew beside a dragon well on a nearby mountain and how the juice extracted from the plant would restore the land to fertility and cure the sick. Many young, brave men from Fujian went up the mountain to find the holy plant but none came back as the well was guarded by a fierce black

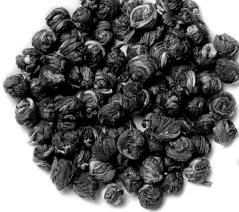

Pai Loong Chu, or white dragon ball tea

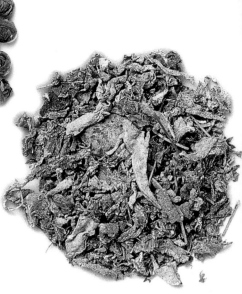

Pai Mu Tan, or white hairy monkey tea

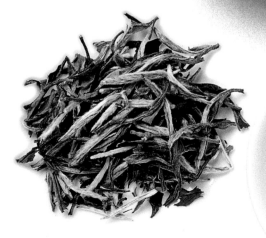

Pai Hao Yin Chin, or silver needle tea

dragon. A family of two brothers and their sister eventually decided they would try and fetch the plant. The eldest brother went first but after 36 days had still not returned. So the second brother set off to try and bring back the holy plant, but after another 49 days he too had not returned. Finally, the younger sister resolved to find the plant and her brothers and set off to the dragon well.

When she arrived she saw that the dragon had turned all the men to stone. Using her cunning she avoided the dragon's magic, reached the well, and slew the dragon with an arrow. She then picked the shoots of the holy plant and watered them with water from the well. They immediately grew into full plants, so she took all the seeds and searched for the rocks that the men had become. She squeezed a drop of juice from the seeds onto each rock until the men were all restored to life. The two brothers and their sister returned to the village and sowed the seeds on the slope of a hill. Immediately they sprang into full blossom. The brothers put the leaves into hot water and let everyone drink, so all the people who were sick became well. Together the family restored the fertility of the land and brought the rains again. From that day, all the plants of Fujian became tea plants and the people of Fujian and their descendants drank the tea.

There is another fairy tale about a white tea called Pai Mu Tan, meaning white peony flowers. There was a young official who could not stand the corruption and bribery in the government so he retired and left with his mother. As he traveled he suddenly became aware of a pleasant fragrance and stopped to ask an old man what it was. The old man told him of 18 peony flowers growing nearby, in the middle of a pond. The man and his mother visited the lake, saw the flowers, and decided to settle there.

One day his mother fell ill. He searched in vain for healing herbs until, tired out, he fell asleep by a tree. In a dream an old man told him that to cure his mother he had to cook a carp with a new tea. He told his mother the dream and was astonished to hear that she had had the same dream. He found a carp and was wondering about the new tea when suddenly there was a clap of thunder and the 18 peony flowers became 18 tea plants. Because the tea plants had been peonies the tea leaves had a white hairy surface. He took the leaves and cooked them with the carp. His mother got better and told him to care for the tea plants. When he agreed she became immortal and flew off, and is now a local patron of tea.

Yellow Teas

Yellow teas are unfermented and get their name from the color of the brew that they make. The tea leaves are yellow but not naturally so: they are deliberately encouraged to become yellow as a by-product of the Stir-frying or Killing Green stage of the tea-making process. Because of the color tone people subconsciously get the impression that the leaves have gone bad so very few people want to drink yellow tea. Some people really like it, for example the Chinese princess in the Tang Dynasty: when she married into Tibetan royalty, she specifically requested that yellow tea leaves be brought with her to Tibet.

However, yellow teas are extremely rare and because they are not sold in shops it is very unlikely you will get the chance to drink them. Mao Chien, Huang Ta Ch'a, and Chün Shan Yin Chin are all yellow teas. Chün Shan Yin Chin is considered the best and the most valuable of all yellow teas.

When infused, yellow teas turn the water a clear yellow-orange color. They have a pure and fresh fragrance and leave your mouth feeling cleansed and refreshed. Unlike white teas, yellow teas have a definite taste, which is quite singular and monotonic. A special characteristic of yellow teas is that their flavor does not change in strength from the time you first make the tea to later when it begins to cool down. It leaves a bittersweet taste on your tongue, especially on the tip. Unlike other teas that make your mouth watery, yellow teas make your mouth drier. It is also possible to detect a slight sourness in the aroma — not in the way that oranges, lemons, or other citrus fruits are sour, but a more herbal sourness, in the way that dates can be sour.

The most famous yellow tea of all is Chün Shan Yin Chin, which was popular during the Tang Dynasty, but rarely drunk now. One of the reasons it is so famous is because when you make the tea the leaves stand vertically: some stand at the surface catching air bubbles while others stand at the bottom of the cup. According to Japanese superstition, tea leaves that stand vertically signify good luck.

According to legend, during the Tang Dynasty a servant was making tea for his king. He was pouring hot water into a cup containing tea leaves when suddenly hot steam came out and a white crane appeared to the king, looked at him, nodded three times, and then soared into the air. Astonished, the king looked back at the cup of tea and saw all the tea leaves stand vertically at the top of the water and sink down, still remaining vertical. He asked the servant what had happened and the servant told him the water came from the white crane lake of Chün Shan and the tea leaves were called yellow feathers. He explained that the crane nodding and soaring into the air meant the king would be prosperous and rise above others. The standing leaves were symbolic of the king's subjects saluting him in respect and when the leaves floated down it signified their yielding to him. Naturally, the king was very happy to hear this. He renamed the tea Chün Shan Yin Chin and drank it regularly. Chün Shan was the place where the water came from and Yin Chin means silver needle. This describes how the leaves stand vertically like needles. The story of Chün Shan Yin Chin also demonstrates the importance of using the right water to make tea: in this case the tea had to be made with water from the white crane lake.

Chün Shan Yin Chin, or silver needle tea, from Chün Shan.

Light Green Teas

There are many kinds of light green teas so it is only possible to make general observations about this group. They are a greenish color with a touch of red, although the tone of red depends on the choice of tea. Light green teas tend to have a wheat-like aroma with a hint of something like wet twigs and grass, and have a salt-like flavor without being salty. They are smooth, strong teas and you will feel a hardening on your lip when you drink them, especially on the front part, as if a layer of skin on your lips is tightening. Light green teas are not dry; indeed, they are very watery and make your mouth secrete a lot of saliva long after finishing your cup. One of the more popular and famous of the light green teas is T'ieh Kuan-yin. "T'ieh" means metal or metallic, and Kuan-yin is the Goddess of Mercy in Chinese Buddhism. A distinct trademark of a good T'ieh Kuan-yin is a white layer like frost on the surface of the leaves. Leaves of wild T'ieh Kuan-yin can also be picked by monkeys (see p. 52).

There are two versions of how T'ieh Kuan-yin came to be named. The first is about a farmer, who was a very faithful Buddhist follower. Every day the farmer made a fresh cup of tea as an offering to the statue of Kuan-yin. One night he dreamed that the goddess came to him and told him of a small tea plant located in a crack of a cliff face. She told him he could take the plant home and grow it so that he and his descendants could enjoy the tea. Most importantly he was not to be selfish and had to share the tea with everyone else. The faithful farmer did as he was told and called the tea Kuan-yin tea to honor her name. The word "T'ieh" was added because the dark green leaves of the plant are heavy and their edges tinged with red like rust on metal.

The second story is about a scholar who, after failing the imperial examination, spent each day climbing the mountains to enjoy the scenery at sunset. One day he noticed a branch growing from a crack in some rocks. So he took the plant home to cultivate in his garden. The plant thrived in his garden and he enjoyed its aroma so much that when he next took the examination he gave the officers gifts of the tea. They too enjoyed the tea and presented it as gifts to higher officers, who were also impressed and in turn presented it to their superiors. Eventually the emperor himself, the famous Chien Lung of the Ching Dynasty, was given the tea. Wanting to know the origin of the tea, the emperor summoned the scholar, who told him that the tea was grown under the Kuan-yin rock and weighed as much as metal. This was how the emperor named it T'ieh Kuan-yin.

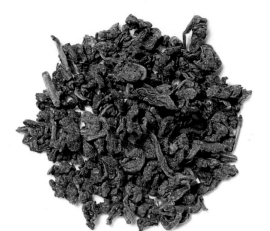

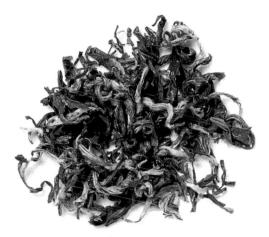

T'ieh Kuan-yin, or metallic Kuan-yin tea. The sample shown here is four years old.

This is an inexpensive T'ieh Kuan-yin tea from Canton, which has a very fresh taste.

Hao Seng tea is easy to find in most Chinese tea shops.

Because T'ieh Kuan-yin tea is quite expensive, some people use other teas, such as Oolong, which also has a reddish edge on the leaves, to impersonate it. Distinctive Oolong tea is famed for its unique aroma and depth of flavor. This variety is indigenous to mainland China, but is so popular that it is now grown in many different regions and countries, notably Taiwan and Japan. In China, Oolong is normally grown on higher slopes, particularly in the southeastern province of Fujian, where it was first found. In Taiwan, Oolong tea is planted and harvested in the mountains, at altitudes of 4,000 feet (1,220 meters) above sea level. This practice dates from the Ming Dynasty when tea planters discovered that the mountain topsoil was ideal for the Oolong tea plant. Because of the early morning chill at such heights, the tea pickers began to associate the Oolong harvest with cold fingers and toes. Eventually, this variety came to be known as Tong Tan Oolong, meaning cold summit Oolong.

The name Oolong dates back to before the Ming Dynasty, when it was still an unnamed bush. One day when the bush was in full blossom a tea planter picked some of its leaves and tried making a tea with them. He drank some and also offered it to his neighbors. His neighbors were particularly delighted with the tea, so the tea planter invited them to name the tea. One morning at dawn, a tea picker saw a black snake silently coiled around a branch of the unnamed bush. When the tea picker drew near, it slid away. Remembering the snake and thinking that it was attracted by the delicious aroma of the tea leaves, the neighbors called the tea Wu-long. "Wu" means black and "Long" means dragon or snake. (In Chinese the same word is used for dragons and snakes.) The name, black dragon tea, has been used ever since, by growers and connoisseurs alike.

Another famous, highly regarded light green tea is Ta Hung P'ao, also known as the emperor of all teas and jewel of all teas. It originates from only four wild tea plants that were found growing on Mo Yi mountain, which is famous for tea making. These plants, two of which still exist today, are the first generation and only produce 7 oz (200 g) of leaves a year. People have taken twigs and cultivated second and third generations of this tea. The second generation

Oolong, meaning black dragon, from Fujian. Although the tea may appear black or green, it is classed as a light green tea.

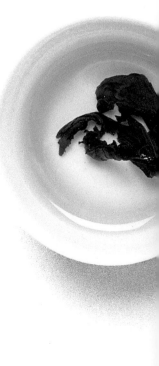

Kwai Shui Kam, or marine golden turtle tea. This very special tea has an unusual taste and is hard to find except in good Beijing tea shops.

only grows 55 lbs (25 kg) a year. The small quantities of this tea available make Ta Hung P'ao an extremely expensive tea, although this not the only reason behind its value: its aftertaste and aroma persist long after drinking it and it is also renowned for its nourishing, medicinal properties. It is said that a local officer of the king fell sick and the doctors could not treat him. The monks of Mo Yi mountain heard of this and brought leaves from the first Ta Hung P'ao plants. The tea restored the officer to health and as a measure of his thanks he hung his red cape, only worn by officers of the king, on the three tea plants. This was how the tea earned its name Ta Hung P'ao, meaning large red cape.

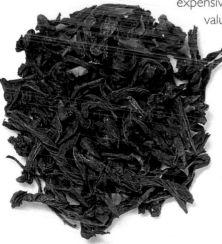

Ta Hung P'ao, large red cape tea.

Green Teas

Green teas are greenish in color with a touch of yellow (the degree of yellow depends on the kind of green tea you are drinking). These teas have a smoky aroma that stays close to the surface of the tea. To smell green tea you have to bring the cup right up to your nose. Green teas also have a fresh, outdoors smell like the scent of early morning mist or damp grass when it has just rained. It has a weak, grassy kind of taste that is quite persistent in your mouth and leaves a roughness on your tongue, rather like when you eat a raw olive.

A famous green tea is Lung Ching, which means dragon well, named after the place where the tea plants are found. Originally, there were only 18 such tea plants and these were grown by an old lady who lived alone in a small village in Hangzhou. Out of kindness to the travelers who journeyed under the hot sun she made tea from the crude leaves, free of charge. One day an old man was passing by and, on seeing her, asked what she was doing. The old lady told him she was poor, alone, and made crude tea for travelers to quench their thirst. The old man said she was not poor at all; indeed, she was very rich and had a treasure within her household. He pointed to the giant stone basin she used for grinding, which contained all her leftover tea sediments. He then offered to purchase it but the old lady told him it was not worth anything and he could take it for free. Because it was too heavy to lift, the old man said he would come back the next day with help and asked if she would keep the basin for him.

The next day when the old man came he saw only a clean stone basin, so he asked what had happened. The old lady told him that she had poured the sediment away and cleaned the basin for him. The old man said it was now valueless as it was the residue of collected tea leaves that was the treasure. He asked the old lady where she had put the tea sediment and she replied that she had sprinkled it over her 18 tea plants and the surrounding soil, so it was not recoverable. However, on that day her 18 Lung Ching tea plants were transformed from poor to top quality bushes.

Yu Ch'ien Lung Ching, or before the rains dragon well tea (see p. 64). This tea must be picked during March before the start of the rainy season.

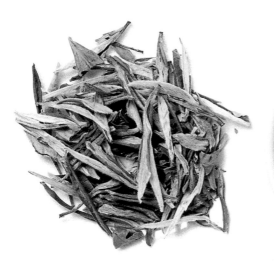

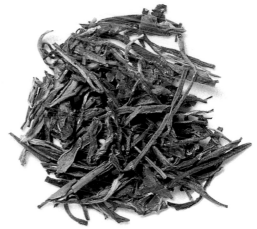

Ho Chin, or pine needle tea.

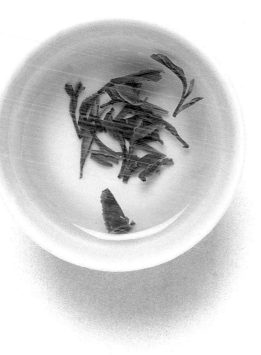

Pi Mo Houn, or white monkey hair tea.

In the second month of the Chinese lunar calendar, normally around March, there is a day that marks the coming of the rainy season. If the leaves are picked just before this day, they make the best of all Lung Ching teas and are called Yu Ch'ien Lung Ching, which means "before the rains Lung Ching." Tea makers often sing a lullaby around this time, which translates as "three days before the rain is a treasure and three days after is grass."

Polee is one of the most commonly drunk teas in the Cantonese community. Its dark, reddish-black color leads some people to think that Polee is a black tea and others to believe it is a red tea, although it is actually a green tea. Polee has been popular since the Tang Dynasty because it can make and serve more tea than other normal teas using the same amount of leaves. It is also popular because it has a strong, persistant aroma and is very good for getting rid of toxins in the body, for helping indigestion, and for removing phlegm from the throat.

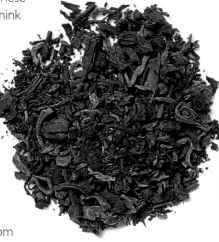

The name Polee comes from the province where it originated. However, it does have nicknames, one of which is K'u Tang. This roughly translates as "pants" tea because, in the past, the lady tea pickers sometimes stole the good-quality leaves from the plantation by putting them into a pouch in their pants.

Even today tea makers prefer to make Polee tea from tea bricks or balls (see also pp. 44–45) rather than loose leaves. It is also well known that the longer you store Polee tea the better the quality. Some of the really old preserved Polee tea leaves are as expensive as the king of teas, Ta Hung P'ao. Some people buy high-quality Polee brick tea for collection and storage rather than for consumption. A number of old Polee tea plants survive to this day, some of which are over 100 years old.

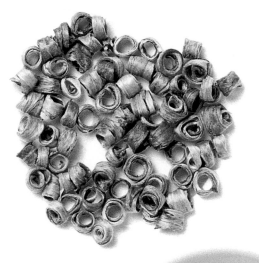

*Left and Right
Four-year-old
Polee tea.*

*Above Yuet Wah Ch'a,
or jade ring tea, is drunk
as a general tonic.
Although this sample is
of average quality, better
types can be expensive.*

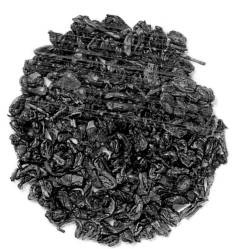

*Above Lo Chu Ch'a, or
gunpowder tea.*

Red Teas

Red teas are dark brown or dark red in tone. They have a very strong, very sharp, and very piercing aroma, rather like baking sweetness. The sharpness of aroma is one distinctive feature of red tea. Another is the fact that, unlike all other teas, its aroma does not fade when you add other elements to the drink. For this reason people like adding extra ingredients to red tea, such as rose, lychee flowers, ginseng, milk, or sugar. Most flower teas have red tea as the base, although there are certain exceptions, such as jasmine teas, which use green tea: green tea brings out the jasmine aroma whereas red tea is so strong it generally covers it up.

Red tea creates a watery effect on your tongue and in your mouth. It also leaves a sandy sensation on your tongue for some time after you have finished your tea. Its taste is very familiar in the West because English teas are all red. Its very distinctive taste seems to disappear immediately after you swallow and it is not until later that you become aware of its very persistant aftertaste.

Ch'i Men red tea originates from the Ching Dynasty and is quite famous in China. The place that it is named after initially made green tea and the story of Ch'i Men tea explains how it came to make red tea. A scholar with the surname Yu was about to go to a big city as a royal official, so his father told him to learn a skill and handicraft which would be useful to him at some time in the future. When he was fired less than three years later, Yu remembered his father's departing words. He recalled that the quality of the green tea his hometown made did not compare with other teas. So he went to Fukien to learn the art of making red tea and when he returned to his hometown he taught his people how to make good-quality red tea.

Red Keemun tea from Keemun province in China.

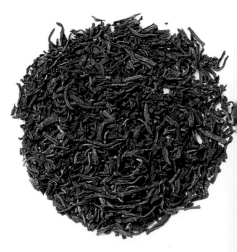

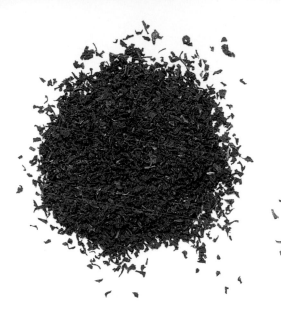

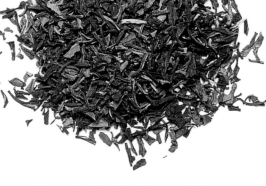

Nilgiri is a fine, fruity red tea with a smooth mellow flavor. It is grown on the Nilgiris, or Blue Mountains, of southern India at altitudes of 3,280–8,200 feet (1,000–2,500 meters).

Darjeeling First Flush has a slightly astringent taste and perfume. Picked only in April, this brown-green leaf tea is from the Tong Song Estate in Darjeeling, northeast India. Darjeeling is sometimes described as the "champagne of teas."

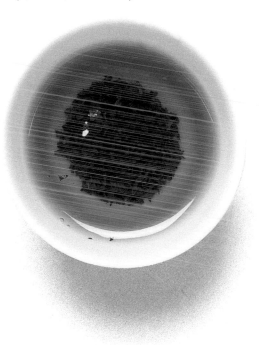

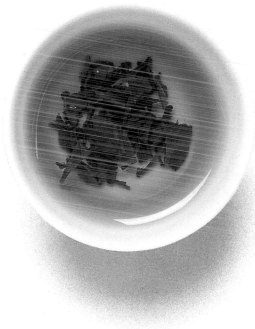

Black Teas

Black teas are not black at all, but make a yellow brew with a touch of green, as opposed to green teas, which are green with a hint of yellow. Black teas also have a dirty appearance. Their aroma combines a bitterness resembling the herbs used in medicine with a metallic dryness, similar to the smell of a heated metal wok.

It is in the taste that black tea lives up to its name: the first couple of sips are extremely bitter, as if you were drinking medicine. With the next few sips the tea becomes bittersweet and as you drink a couple more the degree of bittersweetness changes again. Thus, the distinctive feature of black tea is that the taste changes from mouthful to mouthful. Black tea also leaves a cool sensation in your mouth and a persistent bittersweetness, especially on the back and sides of your tongue.

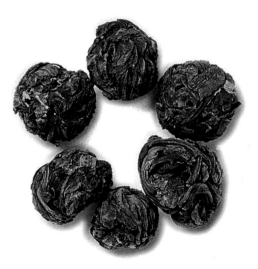

He Lung Chu, or black dragon ball tea.

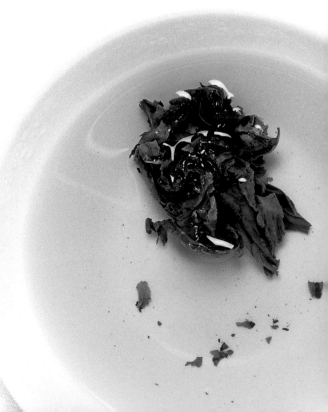

There is a story about a black tea called Wu Tang, or bitter stalk tea. This tea was, at one time, a small production tea and used only as an offering to royalty. Because it was rare and expensive, many people tried to grow the seeds from the plant. They were unsuccessful in their attempts, so they resigned themselves to watching birds eat the seeds. To their astonishment, they noticed that the seeds in the feces of the birds began to germinate. What had happened was that the outer layer of the seed was broken down by the birds' digestive juices, thereby allowing the seeds to grow. Today, growers take cuttings to propagate the plant.

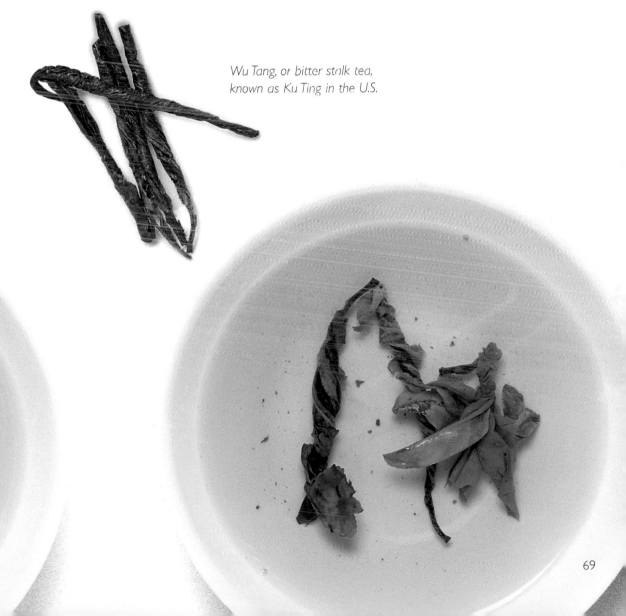

Wu Tang, or bitter stalk tea, known as Ku Ting in the U.S.

Flower Teas

Some teas possess the fragrance of certain flowers and so they are known as flower teas. These teas are named after the flower whose fragrance they possess, for example rose, white peony, and lychee. In these teas, the flowery fragrances are scented into the tea leaves when the leaves are being prepared. The tea leaves can be scented or smoked up to four times — teas scented only once are considered to be of poor quality, while teas scented four times are of excellent quality.

However, it is essential to achieve the correct balance of flowers and tea. If the flower aroma is too strong and dominating, the brewed tea will often have a bitter and unpleasant taste. Equally, if the flower fragrance is too weak, the brewed tea will not be flower tea. As a general guideline, the aroma of a brewed flower tea should be 70 percent tea and 30 percent flower.

Flowers with a strong fragrance would be paired with strong tea and vice versa. For example, flowers such as rose and lychee are paired with red tea while more delicate flowers with a weak fragrance are paired with green, light green, and white tea. Although people like to use jasmine with red tea, the aroma of the red tea tends to overwhelm and dominate the fragrance of jasmine. Jasmine and green tea are a more popular match.

Some enthusiasts of flower teas enjoy the flowery taste so much that they discard the tea leaves and brew the flowers directly in water. However, it is arguable whether these flower waters can be regarded as a form of tea.

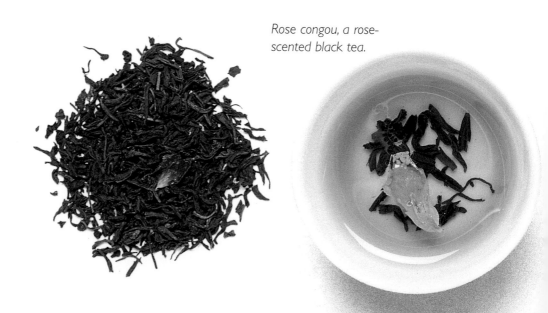

Rose congou, a rose-scented black tea.

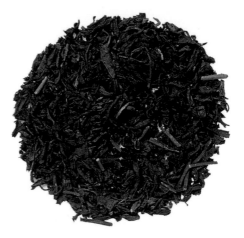

Red tea flavored with lychees.

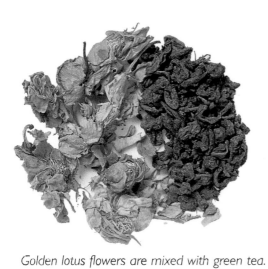

Golden lotus flowers are mixed with green tea.

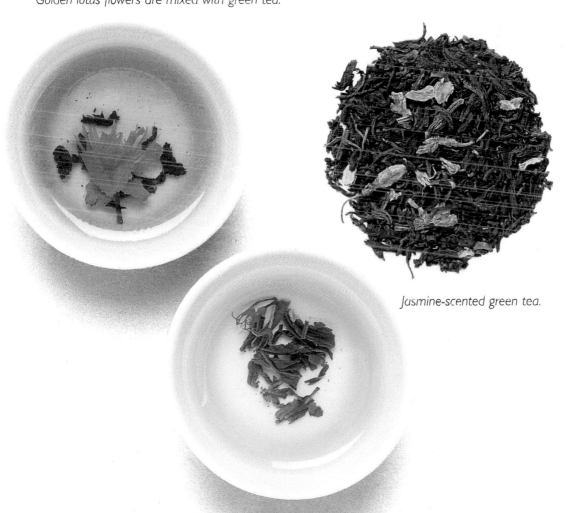

Jasmine-scented green tea.

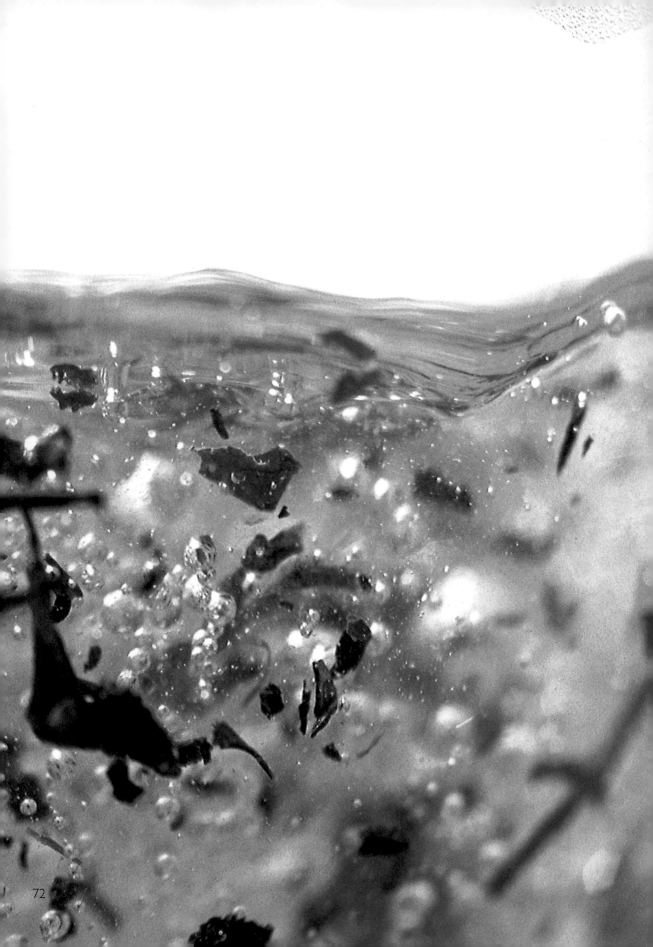

PART THREE

Tea Time

Water, the Mother of Tea 74–76

Heating the Water 77–79

Teapots, the Father of Tea 80- 87

Storing Tea Leaves 88–89

The Art of Tea Making 90–91

Kung Fu Tea 92–111

Water, the Mother of Tea

There are three things that are all important to get the best flavor out of your tea, namely the teapot, the water you use, and how you heat it. In the tea world there is a saying that the pot is the father of tea, water is the mother of tea, and charcoal is the friend of tea.

In the past, the people of China took their water from wells they dug and from nearby streams. Lo Yu, the patron of tea (see pp. 16–18), tells us that the highest quality of water you can use is mountain water, followed by river water, and then well water. The lowest-quality water is from lakes and very deep underground wells. Of all the different kinds of mountain water, the best for tea are said to come from waters that move slowly through stalagmites.

The following story, while exaggerated and probably unfounded, emphasizes the importance of water quality. When they were traveling through the country, Lo Yu and a friend of his, a courtier, reached the famous Yangtse River. His friend said to him, "Since you're such a tea expert, and the Yangtse River is one of the waters you have greatly praised, we must drink tea." Lo Yu looked at the time and replied, "It is now afternoon so the tide and the waves are very strong. It would be too difficult to get water from the middle of the river." However, his friend was very determined to taste the tea they had brought with them, so he sent an officer to fetch the water from the middle of the river. The officer duly returned and presented them with a bucket of water. Lo Yu took a scoop of water from the bucket and examined it and declared, "This is from the Yangtse River but it is not from the middle. It is from the banks and so the quality is lower." The officer said that this was not true as he had taken a boat to the middle of the river.

Silently, Lo Yu picked up the bucket and poured away half the water and then took another scoop of water to examine. Finally, he declared, "This is from the middle of the river and this is the good quality water." The officer, afraid of punishment, turned pale and told them that when he was returning the strong tide had made the boat sway, causing him to spill half the bucket. Thinking it would not matter, he had filled it up again with water from the bank.

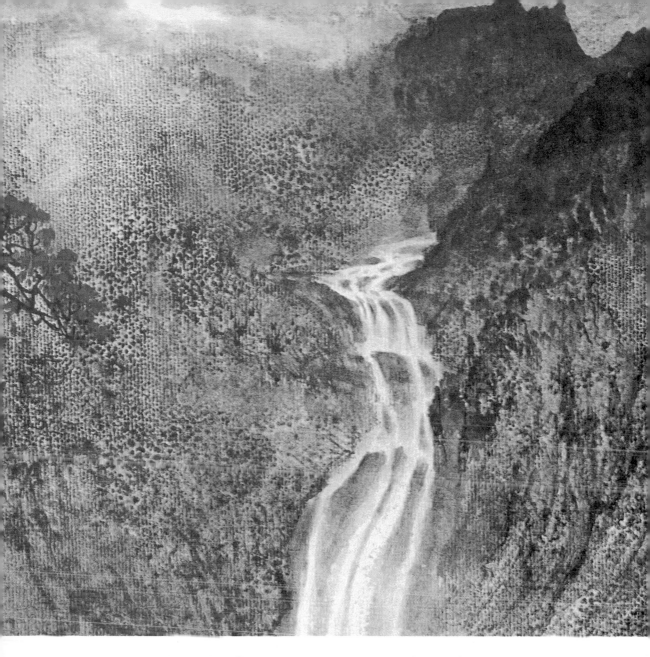

This modern Chinese watercolor celebrates the beauty of water as it emerges from a mountain spring. This is the best water for making tea.

Using the right water for the best flavor

Kin Lung, a famous emperor in the Ching Dynasty, is well known for loving tea as much as life itself. He traveled throughout China tasting every kind of tea and investigating the water that made the best teas. He ordered a silver scoop to be made of a measured unit and requested his subjects to bring to his palace water from all parts of the country. He measured the weight of every sample brought to him and graded them from heavy to light. He observed that the lighter, or less dense, the water the better the cup of tea. His discovery demonstrates the importance of water: the best tea can only reach its full potential if it is brewed with the right water.

Research from the Ming Dynasty further emphasizes this: one tea expert noted that if you brewed tea graded with eight points in water graded with ten, the resulting beverage would have a rating of ten, whereas if you brewed tea with ten points in water with eight points, the beverage would only be rated with eight points. Nonetheless, the best water and best tea do not necessarily make the best possible drink, as the water and tea need to match each other. A simple guide to a good match is to use local tea leaves with local water, as they will naturally complement each other. This is because they share the same soil and mineral composition.

About half of the organic constituents of tea leaves are soluble. Since these are responsible for the flavor, aroma, taste, and coloring of the tea, it makes sense that using the right water will get the best out of the tea leaves. Some constituents are slow to dissolve while others are much quicker. This is why the brewing time is also crucial.

Tap water

In modern society the cheapest and most convenient choice of water is tap water, which can be hard or soft. Hard water is inferior to soft water as it contains more chemical substances. These affect the constituents of tea and therefore impair the taste and coloring of the tea itself. Most tap water is hard, but there are steps you can take to reduce the problem. For example, try using sand or charcoal filters, which are better than chemical ones. Alternatively, let the water stand overnight so that the chemicals fall to the bottom and use only the top half of the water. When the water is heated, use only the top half of the water for your tea. This process temporarily softens the water.

You can use mineral water for making tea but make sure it is one with the least amount of minerals and chemicals. Avoid using distilled water to make tea, for although it is very light, it has lost all of its natural elements and is actually very bad for making tea — far worse than tap water. Hot-spring water is not good for making tea for similar reasons.

Heating the Water

Controlling the temperature of the water is very important when making good tea. The first step is to control the heat produced by the fire. In today's society, unless you live in a rural area, the only option is gas or electricity. If possible, use electricity as the smell of gas will linger in the water.

In the past, to heat their water people used fires that they could fuel with one of three resources available, namely coal, firewood, or charcoal. Coal and firewood both produce smoke that would be absorbed into the water and make the tea taste unpleasant. This is why everyone used charcoal to fuel their fires and also why charcoal is said to be the friend of tea. Professional tea experts prepared their own special fuel. They collected pine seeds or olive seeds, which they dried and burned as fuel. The seeds produced a pleasant fragrance that did not impair the taste of the water. The heat they generated was slow to bring the water to a boil, but because tea drinking was a social event for meeting and chatting, no one minded waiting: they enjoyed the wait and then they enjoyed the tea.

Civil fire and martial fire

In all branches of Chinese cuisine, not just in tea, the role of fire has been recognized and greatly valued. Extensive research has shown that the speed at which the water is boiled and the temperature the water reaches is all important. Chinese cuisine divides fire into two different types, Men For and Wu For, which can be literally translated as civil fire and martial fire. Civil fire refers to the slow, continuous, and lengthy burning of the fuel, while martial fire refers to short periods of high-heat, high-flame cooking.

Martial fire is usually used to control the temperature of the water for tea because civil fire takes too long and overcooks the water. Normally, in China, only fish-eye, or mature water is used to make tea (see pp. 78–79).

Judging the heat of the water

In China, there is a popular folk saying, which can be translated as "The water is boiled, the tea is good." However, this is not true for many teas, as different teas need to be brewed with water of different temperatures. So how can you tell when the water is the right temperature? Chinese research undertaken hundreds of years ago identifies three ways of distinguishing how well the water is heated.

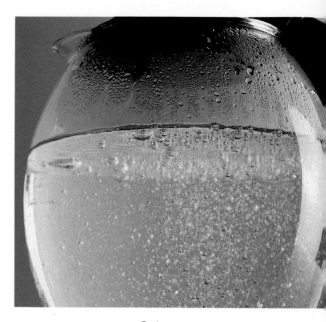

Crab-eye water

The first way is called Sheng Pien, meaning "sound distinguishing." Using your ear you can distinguish three clear levels of heat. At the first level the water makes a low humming sound and is called medium-done, yin–yang, or baby water. Such water is never used for making tea and in fact is never used for anything in cooking, as yin–yang water is said to be unhealthy.

At the second level the water starts to pop noisily in your kettle or container. This is called mature water and is generally the right level for making tea. At the third level, the water bubbles like mad. This is called old man water or white hair water and is not used for making tea.

The second way to judge the heat of the water is known as Chi Pien, meaning "air distinguishing." This involves watching the steam as the water heats up. At the first level the steam rises in small streams, very slowly, gradually, and gently. This baby water is not used. At the second level the steam rises vertically at a moderate volume. This is about the right level for most teas. At the third level the steam ascends at a high volume, like chunks of cloud. This indicates old man water and is no longer suitable to make tea.

The third way is called Hsing Pien, meaning "form distinguishing." This involves looking at the bubbles in the water as it is being heated. At the first level a number of small bubbles come up through the water from the bottom of the kettle or container. Because the bubbles are roughly the size of a crab's eye, this is called crab-eye water. At the second level the small bubbles begin to disappear, to be replaced by continuous streams of larger bubbles. This water is called fish-eye water and is approximately the right temperature for most teas. At the third level the water is bubbling viciously and indicates old man water.

Some teas cannot be brewed with water that is too hot while others can. For example, Polee, Oolong, T'ieh Kuan-yin, and red tea are brewed with fish-eye water, which is about 212 °F (100 °C).

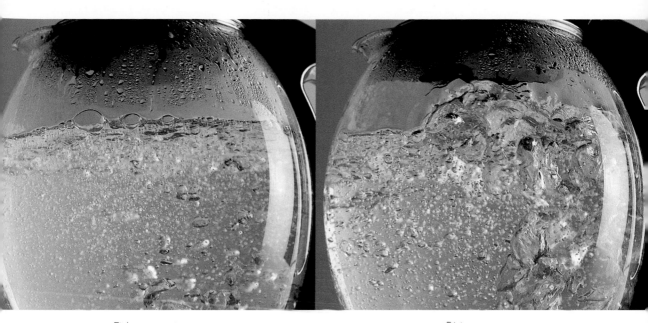

Fish-eye water   Old man water

Delicate teas, such as light green tea, green teas, and flower teas, use slightly cooler water at around 176–185 °F (80–85 °C). To get this temperature, you can either pour the boiled water into a thermos for an hour or you can take fish-eye water, take the lid off the kettle, and leave it to cool down for two minutes. It is important not to use crab-eye water or baby water.

Modern kettles stop automatically when the water starts to boil very rapidly, just as it begins to become old man water. This is acceptable, but not ideal, for making tea.

Metallic chi

In Chinese cuisine the term "metallic chi" refers to the contact of the ingredients with metal. In some cases, including tea making, this is a bad thing. Today, this is more or less unavoidable because people use metal kettles or saucepans to boil water — even plastic kettles have a metal conductor to heat up the water.

Teapots, the Father of Tea

At first there were no teapots in China and people simply made tea in bowls. They heated the water, added the leaves, poured the tea into a container like a rice bowl, and drank it. It was not until much later that craftsmen developed the art of making teapots. Teapots became increasingly sophisticated and, by the end of the Ming Dynasty, craftsmen were producing fine heat-resistant teapots of unsurpassed beauty.

The fact that teapots are referred to as the father of tea stresses the importance of the vessel in which tea is made. There are four main things to consider in a teapot: choosing the most suitable pot, using it to make the best possible cup of tea, taking care to preserve the pot, and appreciating the pot. Appreciating the pot is purely aesthetic and lets you enjoy the craftsmanship and general shape of the pot, the calligraphy and poetry of the writing on the pot, and the beauty of the illustrations. Antique teapots, especially the Ming ones, are highly collectible, as are modern replicas of old teapots. However, the art and appreciation of teapots is a large subject in itself and is beyond the scope of this book.

Materials for teapots

Chinese teapots can be made from several different materials including jade, agate, crystal, lacquer, bamboo, iron, chinaware, sand, and earthenware. Today, for purely aesthetic reasons, teapots may also be made of glass, plastic, and stainless steel. Jade, agate, and crystal are too expensive and not at all practical, so nobody makes teapots from them anymore, while lacquer is no longer popular. The same is true for bamboo, as bamboo teapots affect the taste of the tea and in certain climates eventually change their shape. Iron teapots are no longer made for a number of reasons: their metallic chi makes the tea less pleasant, their conductivity makes them too hot to touch, and they rust easily. Earthenware is regarded as a cheap, low-grade material, so few teapots are made from it today.

The whiteness of chinaware and the fact that it is nonabsorbant makes china teapots easy to decorate and therefore very popular. Also, because china teapots are white inside, you can look to see how strong the tea is when it is brewing. A top-quality china teapot is said to be as white as jade, thin as paper, reflective as mirrors, and make a sound like a "ching" when you flick it gently with your finger or touch it gently with other china. A ching is a sonorous stone used as a musical instrument in China.

Sand pottery teapots come in a variety of neutral colors that make them seem very homey. The Jixing purple sand teapots, which are still manufactured in China, are a prime example of sand pottery and are famous at home and abroad. They are renowned for their unique ability to absorb and preserve the taste of the tea no matter how long you leave the brew standing. Jixing sand teapots can withstand high temperatures and are slow to conduct heat, so that the handle remains comfortably cool even when pouring very hot tea.

Jixing purple sand teapots can be many different colors, as the soil around Jixing where they are made is high in iron and multicolored. Purple sand pottery is also exceptionally strong and an average person could stand on a Jixing teacup without breaking it. Another characteristic of Jixing pottery is the clear, high tone and metallic ring it makes when you touch together two pieces of a purple sand tea set, for example two cups. Incidentally, it is considered rude to try this out on someone else's tea set.

Jixing pottery is unique, as it combines art with practical usage. Jixing used to be one of the main tea suppliers to royalty, which meant that tea experts conducted very thorough research into tea and tea sets. Historically, the craftsmen of Jixing have always taken great care with the calligraphy, drawing, and art on each pot. Their skill is inspirational; indeed, many great scholars have lived in Jixing, composing poetry to celebrate these exceptional teapots.

Choosing your teapot

Ever since the Ming Dynasty teapots have been handmade. Buyers had to know how to recognize the material and craftsmanship used in making a pot. Since they are all different shapes and sizes and without consistent style or quality, choosing a teapot became a skill in itself. For those who wish to appreciate tea today this kind of knowledge is still relevant.

When choosing a teapot for yourself look first at the shape and appearance. This "fateful encounter of the eyes" is very important in Chinese culture — the closest English equivalent is "beauty is in the eye of the beholder." When you look at a number of similar items there is often one that stands out, one that you like on first impression. Follow your instinct and do not buy a teapot you dislike, no matter how good its reputation, because as a constant daily companion it will make you uncomfortable.

In Chinese culture there is no correct or superior way to choose a teapot — it rests with the individual. There is also no rule defining which teapot looks better than another. When you have found a teapot whose appearance you like, open it to smell the interior. No smell at all is good. If you can smell the materials from which it is made, such as china or sand, this is acceptable, but if you can smell anything else, such as oil or a furnace smell, then reject it for making tea. An old teapot, especially an antique one, is good if, after you pour in hot water and let it stand, the water tastes of tea.

Next ask yourself how well the lid fits. The better the fit the better the pot. A teapot with an airtight lid is best, but beware of one that fits too tightly, as the teapot and the lid will get damaged. The best test is to completely fill the teapot with water and then close the lid, covering the air hole on top with your finger. If the water does not come out around the lid then it is a very good pot. If it does then it is not as desirable.

Another important factor is how well the water pours from the pot. If the water chokes, as if it is coming out in lumps, this is not good. What you want is the water to come out in one smooth, continuous, gentle stream. Equally, any backflow of water at the mouth of the teapot or trickling down the spout is undesirable. After you have poured out all the water look inside: if any water remains in the pot this is not a good sign. As a general rule, you want a pot that pours everything out smoothly, gently, and naturally.

You should also consider the handle and check that it is comfortable to hold and lift up. When you pour the water, look to see if it pulls sideways or forward or seems to slip from your hand. If it does, then the weight distribution is not balanced properly. One way of testing a pot to see how evenly the material and the weight are distributed is to place it on the surface of a bucket of water. If the weight is distributed evenly the pot will stay upright; if it tilts one way or another then the weight distribution is poor.

Right The foreground shows a heavily decorated old Jixing pot. The intricately sculpted molding shows a phoenix on one side and a fiery dragon on the other. This decoration is applied over an inner layer of smooth clay. In the background there is a simply shaped, traditional Jixing pot, with matching cups. The cups are quite large and have handles, like Western teacups.

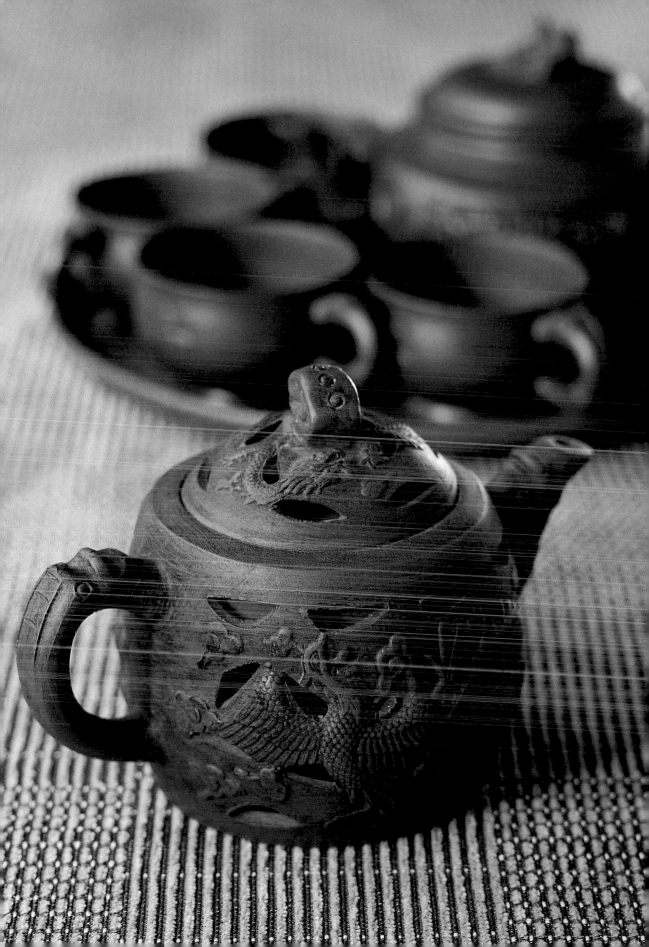

Matching the tea set to the tea

There are two broad groups of tea sets and two broad groups of tea, and a simple test will help you to match them together. Thin, delicate tea sets trap less heat, making them more suitable for delicate teas, namely the green, light green, and flower teas. Thicker tea sets trap more heat and are more suitable for strong teas, such as Polee and T'ieh Kuan-yin. To test your tea set, hold each hand palm up and on each place one piece from the tea set. Bring them together so that they gently touch and make a sound. Don't hold or grab them because your hand will absorb most of the vibration and the sound will be different. The delicate tea sets make a clear, high tone, whereas the thicker sets make a strong, lower tone.

Preparing your new teapot

When you have chosen your teapot, you have to prepare it before you can use it for the first time. This will get rid of any muddy, sandy smell left over from when it was made. Immerse the teapot in a very clean container of cold water and then put the container holding the water and teapot over a low heat. When the water has boiled, reduce the heat and add some strong tea leaves, such as Polee. Bring the water back to the boil and then let it simmer on a low heat for another five minutes. If your teapot is made of water-absorbant material, the amount of time you keep the teapot in the water will affect its color: the longer you leave it in the water the darker the coloring it will aquire. (If you don't want your pot to be a strong color, remove it from the basin after a couple of minutes and let it cool down out of the water.) After five minutes turn off the heat and let the water and teapot cool down naturally. Take the pot out, put it in a dry, dark, cool place and let it dry naturally. Do not put it under the sun, wipe it with a towel or cloth, or put it in a humid place.

Because the essence of a tea will be absorbed into the teapot, tea lovers sometimes have more than one pot for different teas. Some people have several teapots, one for each kind of tea, that is, one for red tea, one for green tea, one for light green tea, and so on. The simplest option is to have two pots: one for aroma-oriented teas and one for the taste-oriented teas.

This is a modern Kung Fu-style tea set made from Jixing clay. The pot is about the size of a man's clenched fist and the cups are about 2 inches (5 cm) wide at the top. Although they appear fine and fragile, the tiny cups are so strong that they can bear the weight of a grown man.

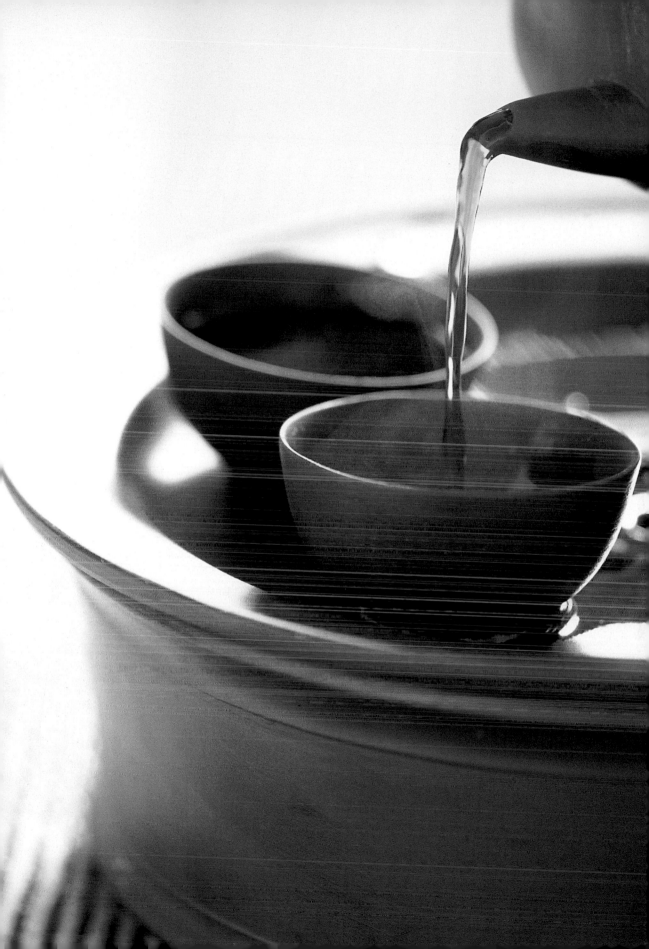

Preserving your teapot

Most tea drinkers do not consider their teapots to be important: they neither care for them nor are particular about how they clean or preserve them. If a teapot is ruined, broken, or lost, they simply go and buy another one. People who care about teas know that their teapots are very important and need looking after. They know that some pots absorb water and will accumulate an essence that assists in releasing the full potential of the next brew. They know that tea sets and this tea essence in the pot can be damaged by bad techniques, such as using dishwashing liquid, powdered cleanser, or even bleach, which many people use for washing their teapots and cups. Some tea sets, such as sand pottery ones, actually absorb the chemicals so that the teapot smells and the tea has a poor flavor and may even taste disgusting.

There are two ways to wash a teapot. The old way, which roughly translates as "a tea mountain within the pot," is not commonly used today because it is considered unhygienic. It simply involves tipping the sediment (used tea leaves) out and making sure that you remove any remaining leaves with the blunt end of a tea needle (see p. 92). You then leave the pot in a dry, dark place to dry. If it has not completely dried by the time you next want to make a pot of tea, you must pour any remaining fluid away first. This old method allows the tea stains to accumulate in the pot so that, as you use it more and more, the tea stain, which can be used medicinally, builds up inside.

A more modern, hygienic way is, after you have finished with the pot, to pour the sediment away, rinse out the pot with hot water, and leave it in a dark, dry corner to dry naturally.

To keep the exterior of the teapot clean and reflective, you need to regularly and carefully wash the teapot with water and gently rub it with your hand — never use anything that will mark or scratch the surface. Pat it dry with a dry cloth. The more you wash the exterior the more reflective it becomes. Don't be tempted to take a shortcut by using oil on an unglazed teapot, as the oil will enter the teapot and damage the essence of the tea inside.

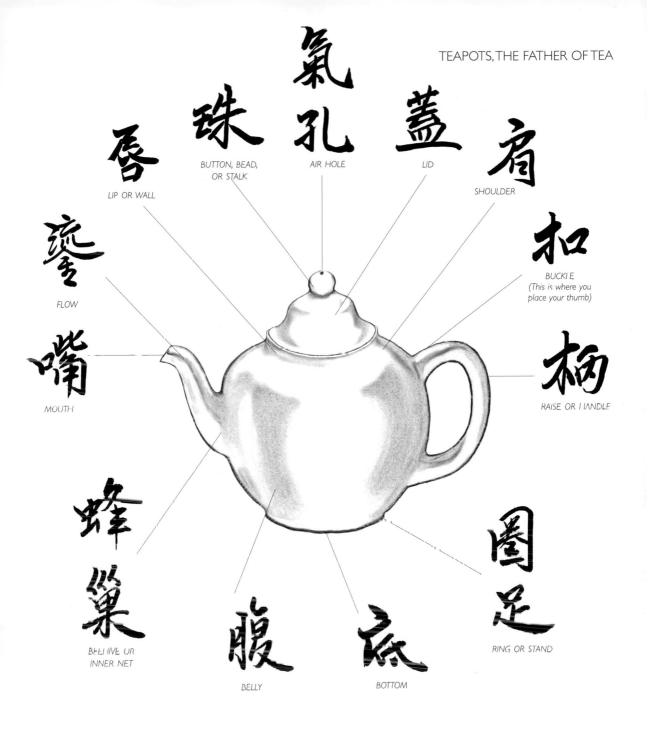

氣
孔 — AIR HOLE

珠 — BUTTON, BEAD,
OR STALK

蓋 — LID

唇 — LIP OR WALL

肩 — SHOULDER

瓷 — FLOW

扣 — BUCKLE
(This is where you
place your thumb)

嘴 — MOUTH

柄 — RAISE OR HANDLE

蜂
巢 — BEEHIVE OR
INNER NET

腹 — BELLY

底 — BOTTOM

圈
足 — RING OR STAND

The Chinese names for the parts of a teapot are extremely specific and for the most part self-explanatory. However, some explanation may be needed for certain parts that cannot be shown clearly in this picture. The lip, or wall, of the teapot lid is the base ring of the teapot lid and allows it to fit snugly and firmly into the neck of the teapot. The beehive, or inner net, is the perforated disc that lies inside the teapot where the base of the spout meets the body of the teapot.

87

Storing Tea Leaves

It is vital to keep your tea leaves dry and away from any humidity that will change their taste. This was crucial in the old days when the supply was small and people could buy only once for the entire year. It is still quite important now as good-quality tea leaves are still only harvested once a year. Some teas are purchased and stored for 10 or 20 years, because the older they are the better they are, like certain wines.

Tea leaves are extremely dry and so are liable to absorb water and any chemical or odor from the air. If the tea leaves come into contact with water, they will rot and a high heat will turn them yellow and make them bitter. Leaves should not be stored next to anything with a strong or pungent smell, such as pepper, curry, or chili, or be exposed to sunlight or air. For this reason, glass or plastic containers and paper bags are not suitable. The best and most common way to store tea is in an airtight aluminum container. You can use a foil container or other airtight container, but don't use chinaware or plastic containers: the former will not be airtight and the latter will make the tea smell.

If you buy a large quantity of tea leaves, use two containers, one large, one small. Store the bulk of the tea in the large one and keep the small one for everyday use, filling it up from the larger one. When refilling the small container use a scoop, not your hand, as the leaves will absorb sweat and smell of your skin. It is also important not to stuff or compress the leaves in either container. Let them have space and be loose, otherwise you will crush the leaves and turn them to dust. Be careful where you store the large container and make sure it is not in the kitchen where there is lots of steam, different smells, and heat. Also, you must never store two kinds of tea in the same container, even if you separate them with a divider, otherwise the leaves from one will absorb the aroma from the other and will aquire a strange aroma and bitter taste.

Right The shiny aluminum container in the foreground has an ingenious upper compartment for storing a small quantity of tea. This allows the rest of the tea to remain in darkness in the lower compartment. The colorful cylindrical containers behind it are made from dense cardboard and lined with aluminum foil. These are also good for storing tea and are much cheaper. The curvaceous brown pot is also made from aluminum but has a bronze-like finish. The narrow neck prevents too much light from getting to the tea when the lid is removed.

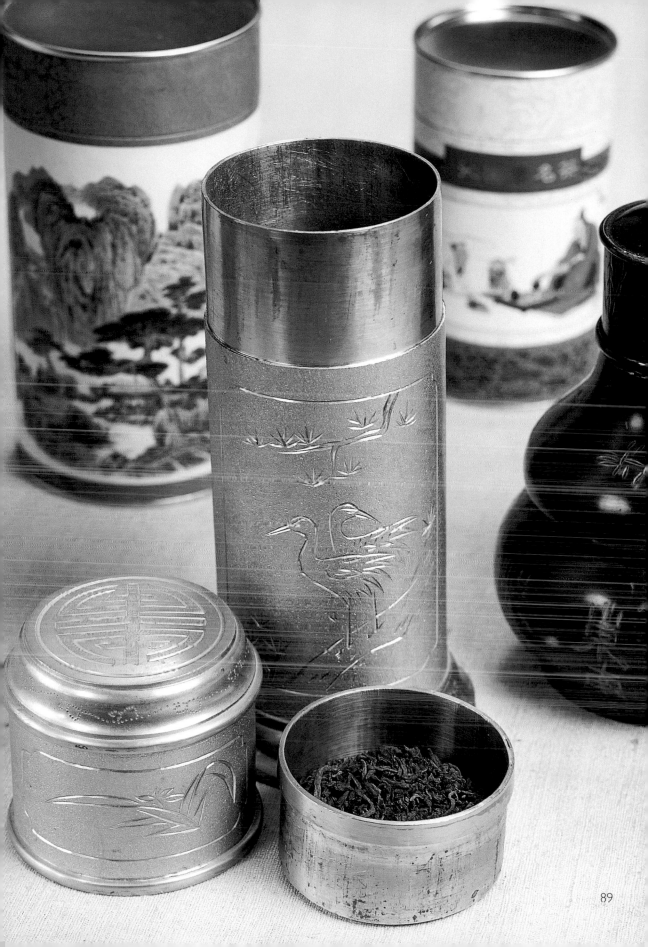

The Art of Tea Making

Originally an outdoor pursuit, tea making in China was an informal affair. All that was needed was a good fire, fresh — preferably mountain — water, a vessel for boiling the water, tea leaves, and a bowl to pour the tea into. It was a joyful, picnic-style occasion that typically followed a long day's work or walk in the mountains. People would make a fire, collect the water from a nearby spring or waterfall, and gather around the fire to make the tea. Over the years the Chinese imperial court adopted the custom of drinking tea. They drank it in the ornamental gardens or in special small buildings dedicated to making and serving tea to family or friends. In the cities, pavilions for taking tea became meeting places and were visited by men who would talk politics or business or simply relax. Special equipment was developed, culminating in the decorative pots and cups that we see today. Taking tea became a formal process and different styles of making and drinking tea developed. Some of these special traditions remain today.

One such tradition is to tap on the table and there is a story behind this. An emperor was concerned about the living conditions of his subjects and wished to see for himself what life was like outside the court. He dressed as an ordinary man and, taking a few guards with him, also dressed in ordinary clothes, went to a tea pavilion in the town. He asked for tea, and a pot of tea with cups was brought to the table. The waiter poured the tea and set the pot beside the emperor. When they had drunk the cups of tea, the emperor served more tea to his men. The men needed a secret way to show their gratitude and respect to their emperor and, using two fingers, his guards bent their knuckles and knocked them on the table. This was to signify kneeling before him. A reference to this tradition survives today: when your host pours you a cup of tea you should tap your first two fingertips twice on the table as thanks.

Making and serving the tea

The first vessels used for drinking tea were big bowls, hence the name big bowl tea. The tea was brewed in the water kettle and poured into the bowls, from which it would be sipped. Tea is still made and drunk in this way in some rural districts of China. The next development was a tea bowl with its own lid and saucer. As serving tea became more formal, a larger lidded bowl was used as the teapot and the tea poured into separate, smaller cups. Because of the proliferation of pots, a much larger bowl-shaped tray was provided to contain both pot and cups. Later, both these were made more elaborate, with a handle and spout, which made them easier to use. The handles also allowed ladies of the court to look elegant during the tea ceremony — previously, their elbows stuck out in an ungainly fashion when they poured and drank tea, as they had to use both hands to hold the tea bowl. This was considered most inappropriate.

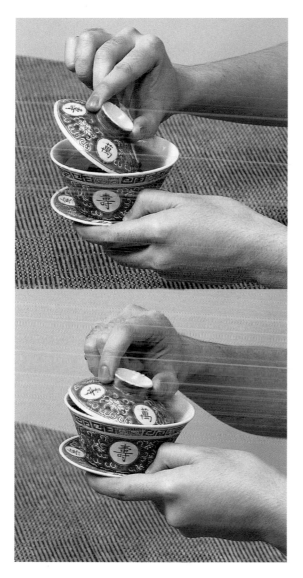

Left This modern, old-style tea bowl is decorated as many such tea bowls were 100 years ago. It is not as large as a "big bowl" and has its own lid and saucer. Any tea leaves floating on the surface of the water are pushed away with the lid.

Bottom Keep the lid in position as you bring the bowl to your lips to sip the tea.

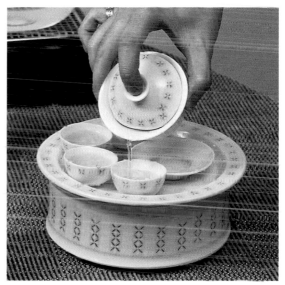

Above This is a modern set of Kung Fu-style tea bowl and cups, complete with perforated draining tray and larger bowl in which the tea bowl and cups are both stored and carried. The decoration is modern.

Kung Fu Tea

As fine teas were developed, a very formal ceremony of taking tea grew up. Different kinds of rare and expensive quality teas were appraised and enjoyed using special small, very fine pots and cups. Today, these tea sets are called Kung Fu tea sets. Kung Fu has two meanings in China: the first describes the martial art, the second means lots of work.

The Kung Fu tea ceremony is a very refined way of drinking tea and a speciality of Fukien. Historically, Fukien is the major tea-producing town in China and even today tea produced in Fukien is exported for national and international consumption. Normally, the host would make a very strong brew and it was not uncommon for the little pot to be half-filled with tea leaves. When making Kung Fu tea today you can of course choose how strong to make your tea.

The following pages show the art of making Kung Fu tea. The movements are extremely refined and flowing, yet precise. They are designed to produce a perfectly brewed cup of tea. Don't be daunted, as the whole process from boiling the water to serving the first cup will only take about10 minutes; experienced tea makers will take only 5 minutes .

For strong teas, such as red or black tea, keep the water at 212 °F (100 °C); for lighter teas like green or flower tea, keep it at 176 °F (80 °C). Once you have boiled the water, a small table plate warmer will keep it at the right temperature. It is important to pour all the water off the tea leaves each time you pour a brew.

Right This modern Jixing tea set is arranged on a new wooden tray, which is perforated to allow water and tea to drip through into a large hidden plastic tray. Trays such as this one can be made from stone, wood, or plastic, and painted or sculpted with images of Buddha, dragons, birds, flowers, or calligraphy.

The cylindrical bamboo vase contains three bamboo tools, a scoop (the tea must never be touched by hand or the delicate leaves may absorb the skin's scent or impurities), tongs for lifting the tiny cups, and the tea needle. The tea needle has a long point at one end and is blunt and spatulate at the other. The point is used for clearing any leaves that may enter the spout and interrupt the flow of tea. The blunt end is used for scraping leaves from inside the pot when the tea is finished.

The small, carefully folded towel is used to wipe the bottom of the pot before pouring the tea. Fresh tea leaves are stored in the curvaceous, bronzed caddy.

1 Washing the pot

Set up the tea set and boil the water.

Completely fill the pot with water and replace the lid.

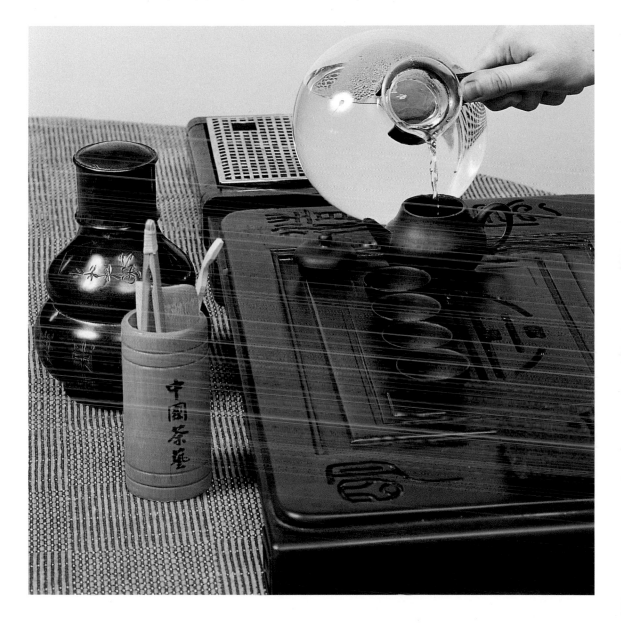

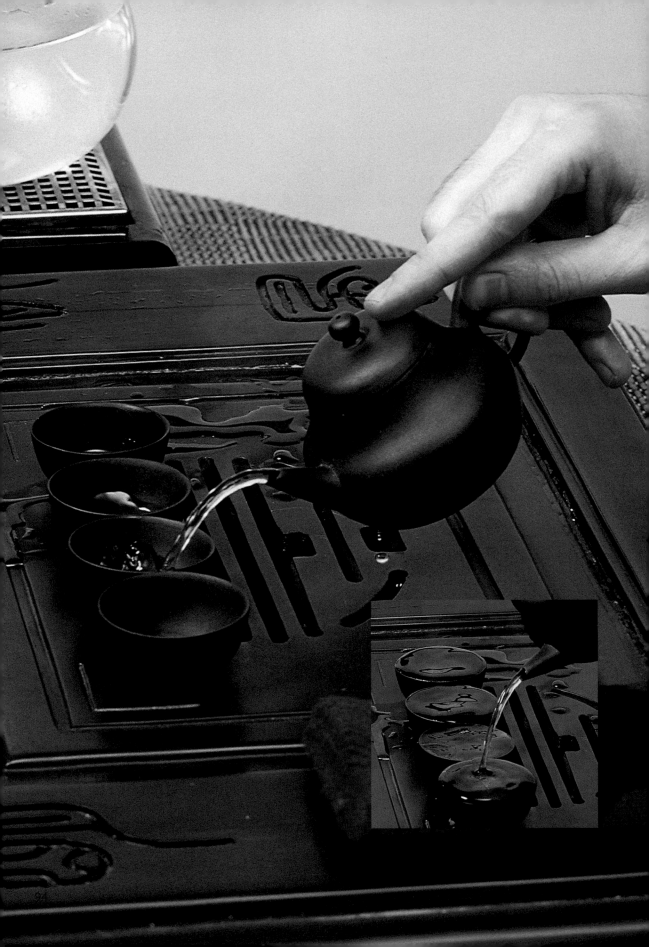

2 Washing the cups

Now pour the hot water in a gentle, continuous stream into the tiny cups.

Starting at one end of the row, move back and forth until all the water in the pot is used. It is crucial to master the swift, flowing movement. This is the action of pouring the tea and you can practice it now while washing the cups.

Notice that there is a particular way of holding the pot. Place your forefinger firmly on the lid to keep it in place.

Using the bamboo tongs, pick up the first cup and tip the water into the second cup, allowing it to spill over the sides. Now gently rotate the first cup around in the water-filled second cup until both the inside and outside have been rinsed.

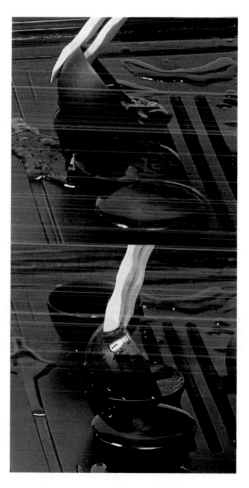

Continue working down the row of cups, washing each one carefully. When you finish, tip the remaining water through the draining holes in the tray.

Now both pot and cups are fresh and warm, ready for the next stage.

Tea masters will complete this cup-washing process in the twinkling of an eye, by using tongs in each hand!

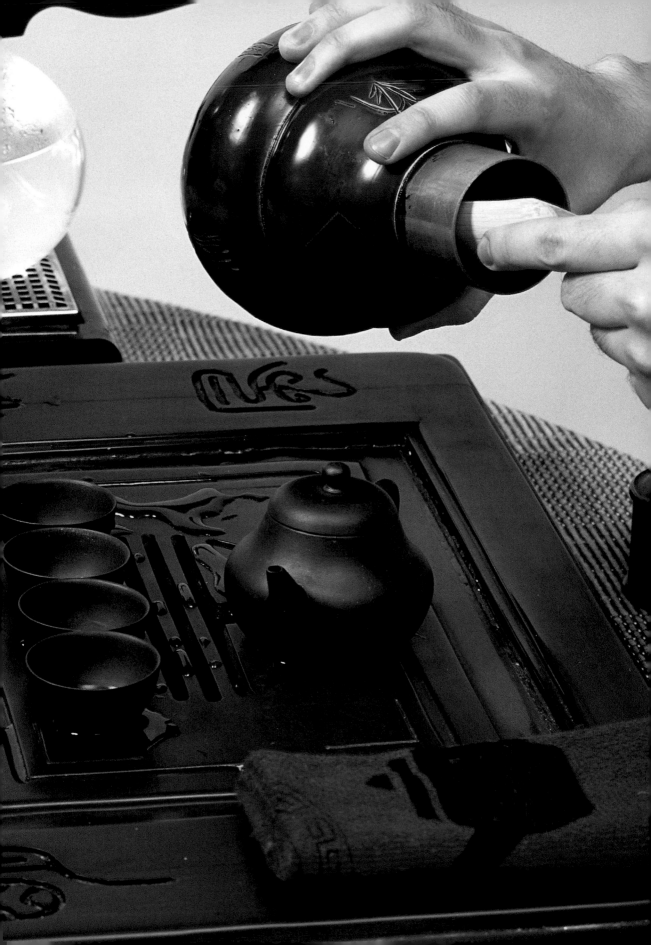

3 Showing the tea

Historically, T'ieh Kuan-yin tea is served from Kung Fu tea sets. However, for the Kung Fu style of taking tea, special teas will be used. You may have spent a great deal of money on the tea. Some special teas can sell for $750 a pound. Special or important guests will be very pleased to inspect the tea leaves. Or you may have a series of different teas, all of which your guests will like to look at before the serious business of tasting begins.

Now for the tea!

Using the bamboo scoop, measure out the tea leaves.

Show the leaves to each guest in turn, starting with the most senior.

Once the tea has been inspected and its color and form discussed, you may tip the leaves into the clean, warm pot.

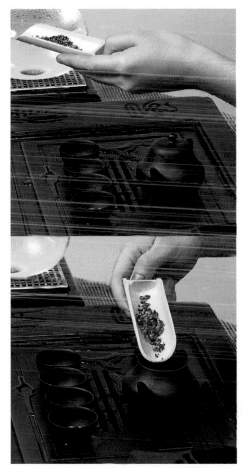

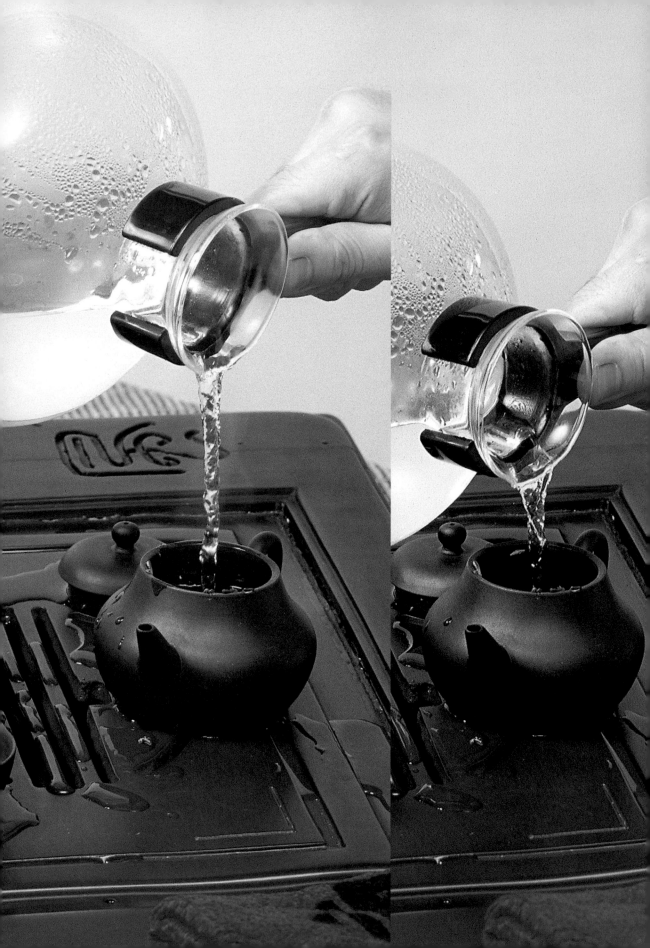

4 Washing the tea

In Chinese culture, the heart is considered the center of love, and the gall bladder the center of courage. It is important to avoid breaking the courage (gall) of the tea.

So, begin by pouring the boiled water around the inner sides of the pot. The tea heaped in the center can gently absorb a little water first and not be swamped right away. This is described as not frightening the tea.

Don't pour the water from too great a height, as it will cool too much and absorb too much air.

Now pour into the center of the pot, moving the water kettle up and down through the air three times. This up and down movement is regarded as a sign of respect, like three welcoming bows to your guests.

Fill the pot right to the brim and replace the lid.

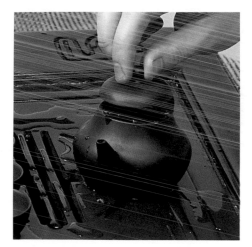

5 Foot water

This washing of the tea produces a lightly tinted liquid which in Chinese slang is called "foot water" — like the water you wash your feet in, it is not suitable to drink. The tea leaves, which have been so lovingly prepared, cooked, and dried, have never been washed until now! The water you have poured onto the leaves will have dust specks and impurities floating on it, so throw it away.

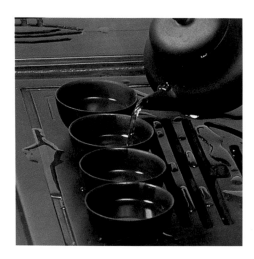

Very quickly pour the foot water into the little cups, again practicing the graceful back and forth movement. Pour all of the foot water from the pot.

Now, using the bamboo tongs, pick up each cup in turn and empty the foot water through the holes in the tray. Do this as quickly and smoothly as possible.

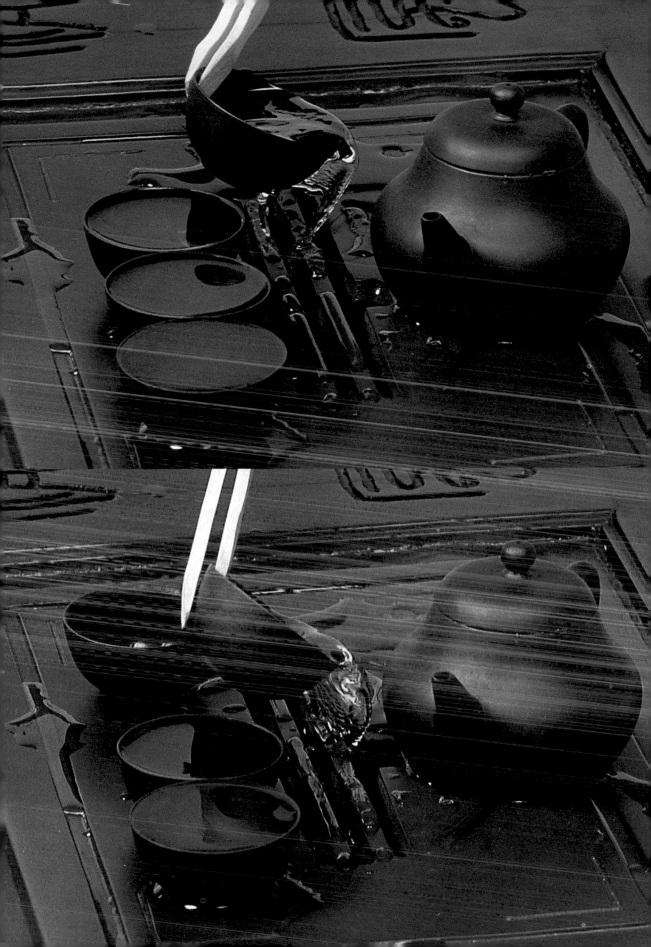

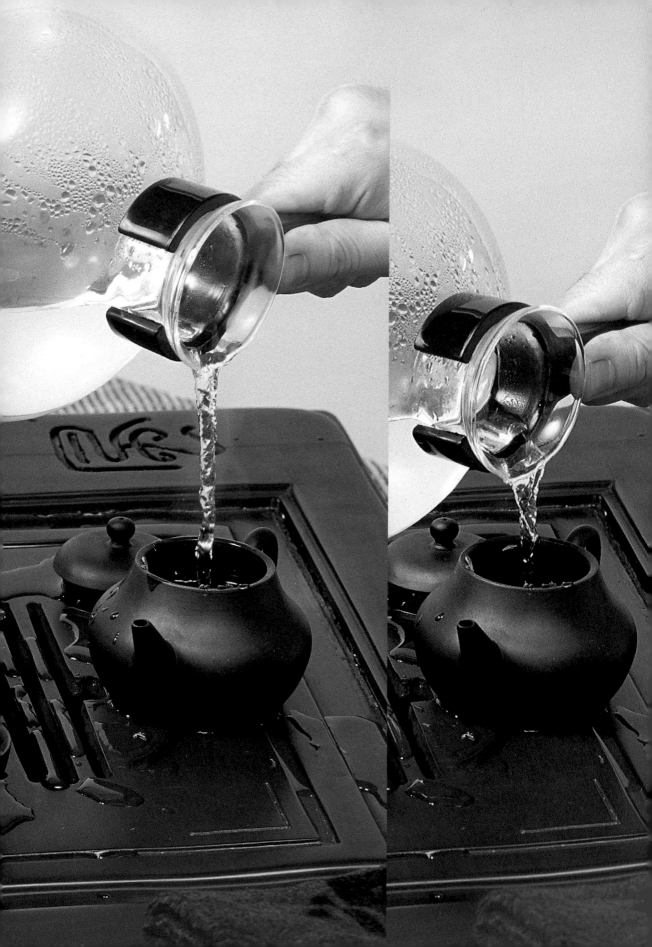

6 Making the tea

Immediately pour fresh boiled water onto the washed tea leaves in the pot.

As before, start by pouring around the inner edges of the pot in a gentle, continuous stream and then into the middle, up and down three times until the pot is full to the brim.

Replace the lid and pour water over the outside of the pot. This will both clean the outside of the pot and make it nice and hot.

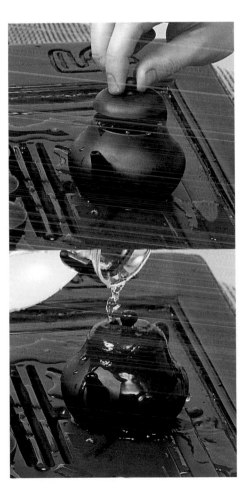

7 Pouring the tea

This is the third time of pouring. You poured first in order to wash the pot and cups; second to discard the "foot water." Now you will pour the first brew of tea.

The purpose of this style of pouring is so that each cup of tea tastes the same and is the same temperature. If the cups were to be poured one after the other, the last cup would be stronger than the first

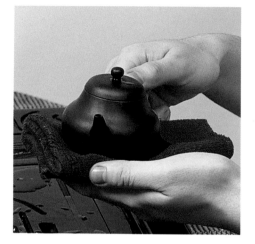

You have just washed the pot. Most of the water will have evaporated from its hot surface. Pick up the pot and gently wipe its base with the folded towel. Replace the towel and start to pour.

Starting at one end of the row of cups, swiftly pour back and forth into each cup. This sweeping, pouring action must be done in one continuous stream until the cups are filled.

Do not fill the cups completely or they will be hard to handle. If any tea remains in the pot, pour it out through the draining holes of the tray.

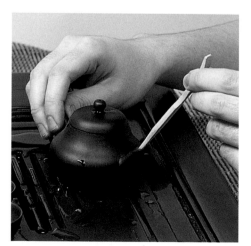

If the flow of tea from the spout is interrupted during the pouring, take the tea needle from the bamboo vase and poke the pointed end into the spout to clear the blockage before continuing to pour.

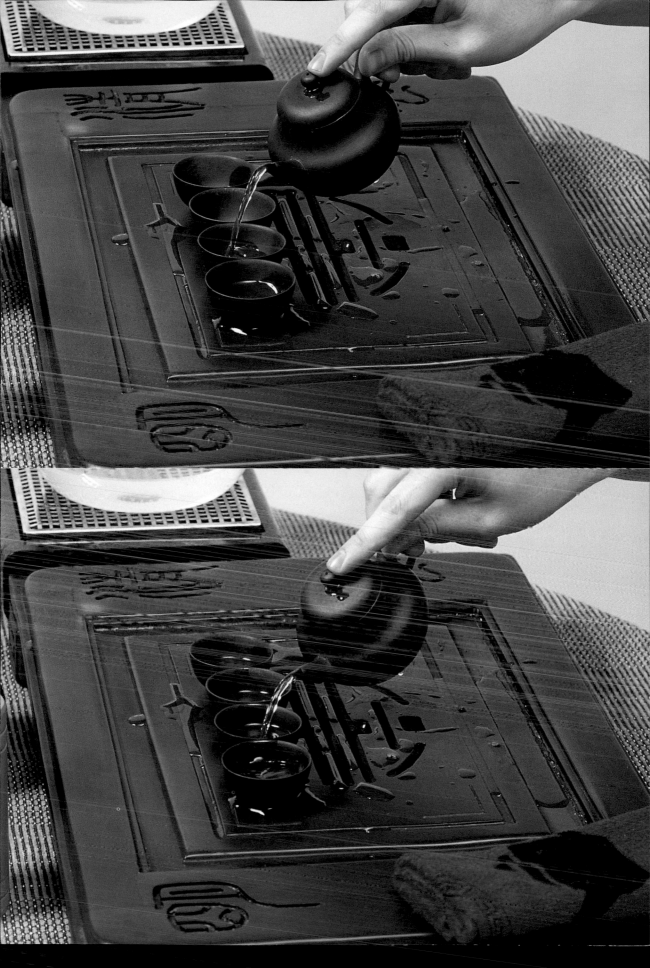

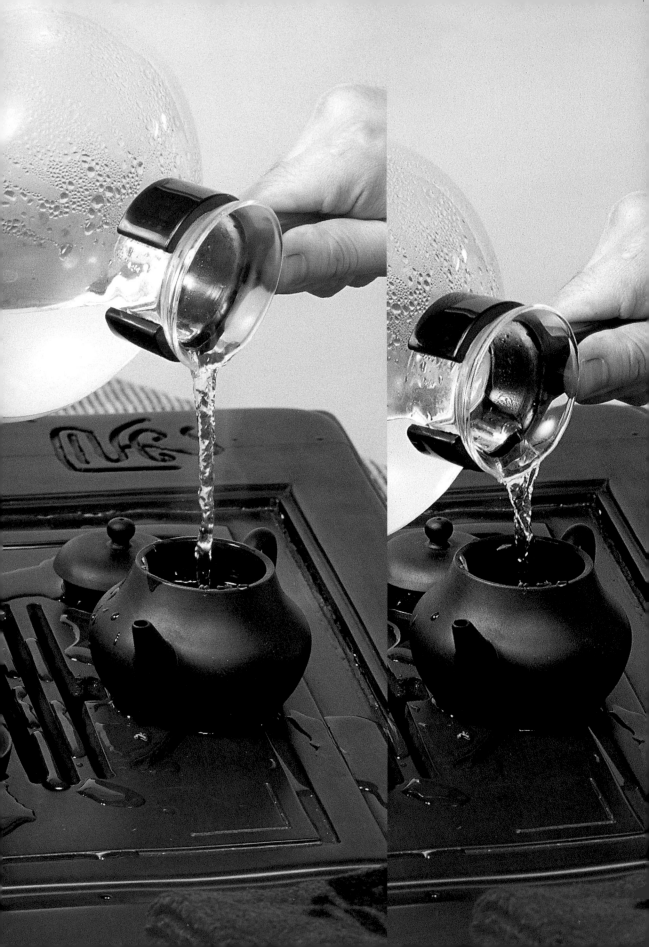

8 Making the second brew

You must make the second brew of tea before serving the first.

Depending on the type of tea, the length of brewing time can vary from 2 to 5 minutes.

Quickly pour more water onto the leaves in the pot. Don't forget the up and down movements.

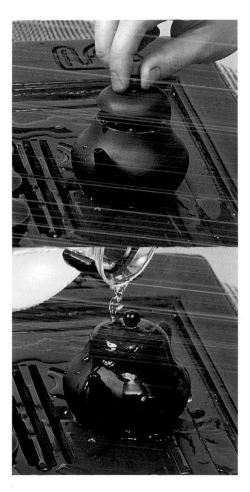

9 Serving the tea

Now you are ready to serve the tea. There are two ways of doing this.

The formal way is to gently pick up a cup of tea, using both hands. It is good manners to always use both hands when serving. Offer the first cup to your most senior guest (using one hand as a tray and the other to hold the cup between thumb and forefinger). Your guest will respond by stretching out both hands to receive the cup.

The less formal way is to make a graceful sweep with your hand, indicating that your guests should each take a cup. The correct way to hold these cups is with just the thumb and forefinger.

Your guests will admire first the color of the tea, then its fragrance before enjoying the flavor.

As the cups are so small, your guests will quickly drink the tea and replace their cups on the tray so that you may pour them fresh tea from the second brew. Tea may be brewed up to 3 or 4 times using the same leaves.

If you are serving another, second type of tea, you will wait for half an hour before doing so. The used tea leaves may be kept and used for other purposes (see p. 139). The teapot and cups are then washed and the whole tea-making sequence repeated. Or a new tea set may be used for the new tea.

During this time, tea snacks or "dim sum" may be served.

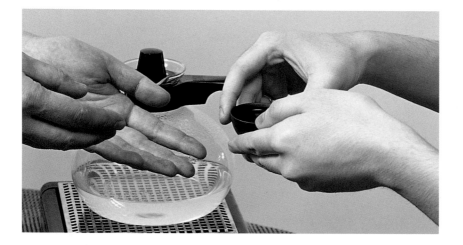

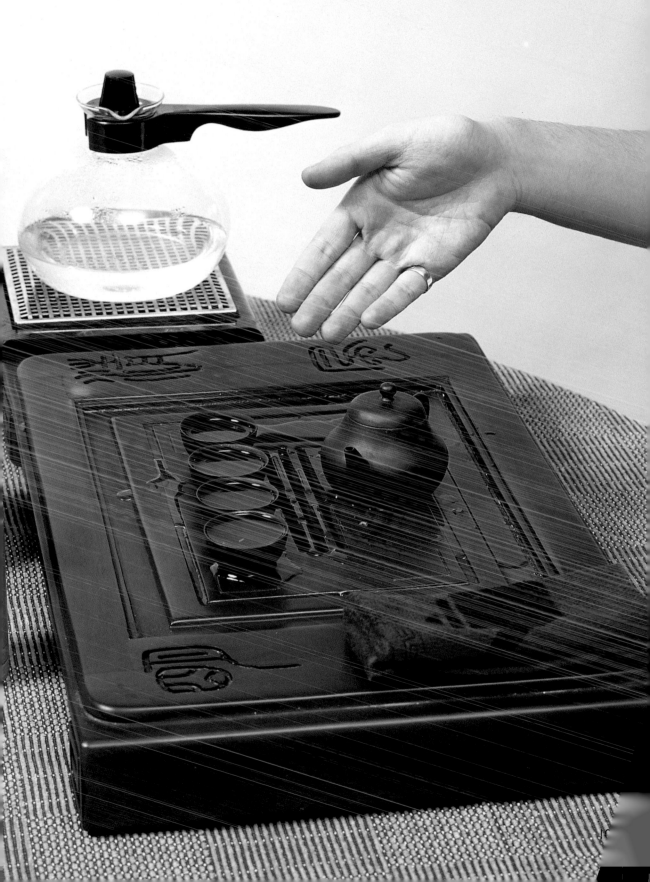

Using a bowl set

This more traditional style of tea set has a large bowl called a tea boat in which the teapot and cups sit. It also has a jug called a tea ocean. The jug is for pouring excess tea into. There is also a set of little tray-like saucers on which to stand the cups.

Fill the pot with boiled water and pour it out into the cups. Using tongs, rinse each cup in the adjacent cup and discard the water into the bowl.

Measure the tea leaves into the pot and pour water in a continuous, gentle stream — start around the inner edges of the pot and then into the center, lifting and lowering the pot three times. Pour this "foot water" off into the cups and then discard it. Pour water onto the leaves in the pot as before. Fill to the brim, replace the lid, and pour water over the outside of the pot.

Lift the pot and pass the base around the rim of the large bowl. This motion stirs the tea leaves.

Wipe the base of the pot with the folded towel.

Pour the tea in a continuous stream, moving quickly back and forth so that each cup of tea is of equal strength and heat.

Pour excess tea into the jug.

Place each cup onto a little boat and hand it to your guests. There is no need to make more tea immediately as you have the small jug for second helpings.

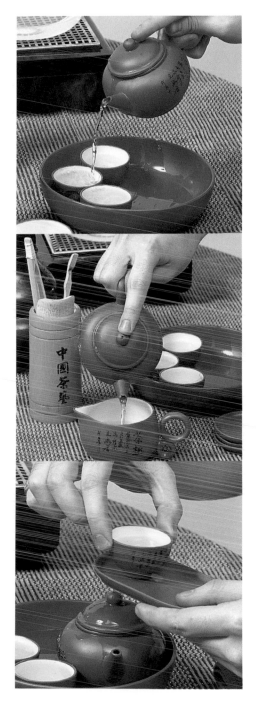

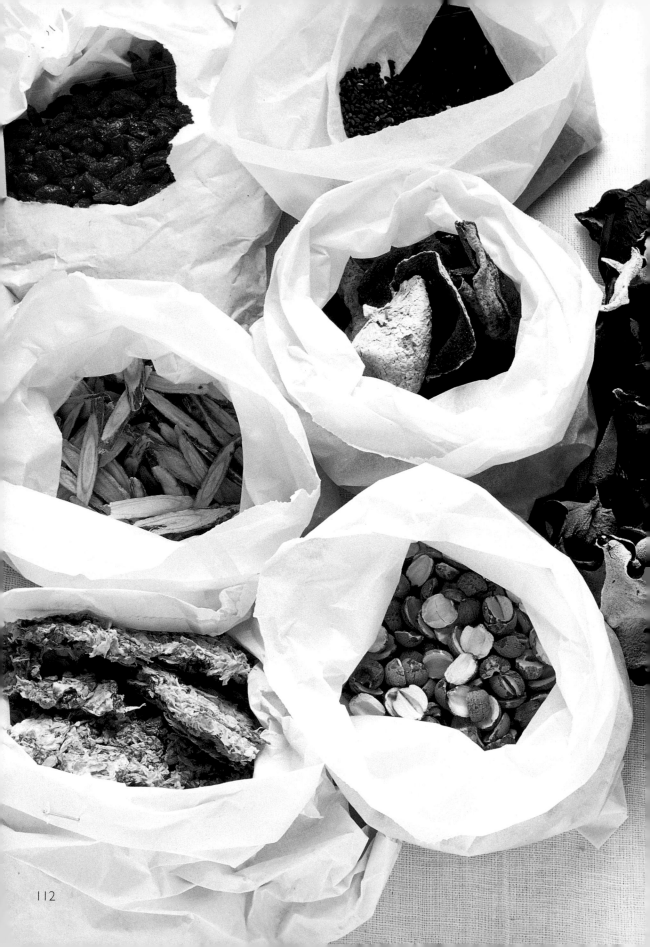

PART FOUR

Healing Teas

A Culture of Health 114–117

Introducing the Healing Teas 118–137

Cautions and Uses of Tea 138–139

A Culture of Health

The cultivation of good health has always been central to the Chinese, one of the most enduring civilizations in human history. Their medical model is based on a fundamental understanding of the body's energy patterns. This understanding, although ancient, is strikingly similar to some of the latest discoveries in Western contemporary science.

A traditional Chinese doctor views each aspect of a person, from bones to brain waves, as a manifestation of an all-pervasive life force, or "chi." A healthy person is someone whose chi flows smoothly and without obstruction throughout his or her being. Pain, infection, and illness are attributed either to blockages in the free movement of energy or to a weakness in the energy field, resulting in vulnerability to the external influences that cause health problems. According to Chinese medicine, the mind and body are also so closely interlinked that mental tensions can produce internal energy imbalances and lead to physical disorders. For this reason, a person needs to be inwardly warm and relaxed to remain healthy. In this model of interacting energies, our external environment has an unmistakable effect on us, body and mind. Therefore, in order to withstand attacks from hostile energies, a healthy person needs a sympathetic environment and physical and mental strength.

Naturally, anything that promotes the smooth flow of energy, overcomes internal blockages, warms and relaxes us, and fosters a positive environment will help a person stay healthy. This is exactly what tea offers: a warm cup of tea is a positive source of energy and its combination of warmth and fluidity stimulates the flow of a person's chi and improves its circulation throughout the body. The properties infused into the water from the tea leaves also refresh the mind, and a lively, alert mind is one of the keys to health: a sluggish mind dampens down the flow of chi, whereas a vibrant mind stimulates it.

In China, tea is regarded as one of the main aids to a long and healthy life. Tea that is made the right way and is not too strong or too weak, combined with daily excercise, can keep your body healthy all your life. This is because it refreshes a person's body and spirit and promotes energy. In remote mountain areas people often live for over 100 years. There they drink the best tea, which grows at high altitudes and is gathered and made by local people, using pure mountain water.

Right Drinking tea and sharing dim sum at a busy restaurant in central Hong Kong.

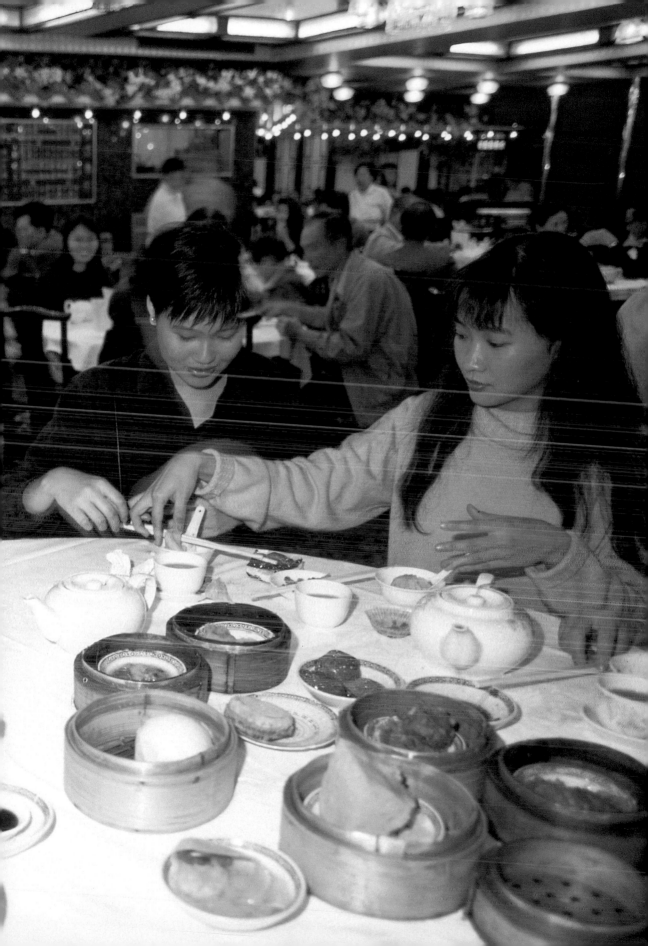

It is not surprising that teahouses have been so popular across the Chinese-speaking world. Throughout the changing seasons, tea acts as a natural thermostatic regulator: in cold weather, a hot cup of tea is ideal for helping the body to keep warm, while in hot weather, warm tea is the drink that will cool you down most efficiently. This is because it gently raises the body temperature, thereby encouraging the body to sweat and cool itself naturally. Even though the idea of quickly drinking large quantites of chilled beverages may be appealing, it creates a lot of disturbance in your body and subjects it to stress, rather like throwing a stone into water. It could also be likened to throwing water onto a fire, for although the water produces quantities of steam, it actually increases the flame.

Possibly the most important characteristic of tea is its ability to relax the drinker. Traditionally, people take time off for tea. It is a time to sit with others, either to enjoy a period of repose or to chat with friends. When freshly brewed tea is poured from the teapot, it is normally too hot to drink. This is a wonderful opportunity to sit back, relax, watch the steam from your cup coil into the air around you, and allow the aroma to fill your nostrils. As you wait for the tea to cool down, the tensions of the day will slip away unnoticed. Tea is a silent but powerful influence in our lives.

Medical science and tea

In terms of modern medical research, it has been proved that tea possesses a wealth of health benefits. Drinking three to four cups of mild, good-quality tea each day can provide protection from all kinds of ailments. Scientific examination of tea has shown it to contain a cocktail of health-giving constituents, such as vitamins B1, B2, and B6, as well as vitamin C, flavonoids, and polyphenols.

Tea is also rich in two key minerals, namely manganese, which is essential for bone growth and body development, and potassium, which helps to keep the heart beating and maintain the fluid levels in the body. Tea is also tooth friendly, as it is one of the few natural sources of fluoride. Oral hygienists increasingly believe that tea improves overall oral health by preventing tooth decay and reducing plaque.

There is growing scientific evidence that the antioxidant effects of the flavonoids in tea are important in helping to prevent cancer of such organs as the pancreas, prostate, colon, esophagus, and the mouth.

Antioxidants work by preventing and repairing free radical attack in the body. Of equal significance is tea's ability to combat heart disease and reduce the risk of strokes: studies show that tea reduces blood cholesterol and blood clotting and lowers blood pressure. Perhaps the most striking development in medical research has been the recent assessment by staff associated with the Harvard Medical School. They found that a person who drinks a single cup of tea a day can cut the risk of having a heart attack by 44 percent. This is due to the powerful antioxidants in tea, which counteract fatty deposits in the arteries. In short, a good-quality tea can help to keep down cholesterol and improve circulation by helping to increase blood flow and prevent hardening of the arteries.

Another study showed that men who drank green tea burned up more calories than men who did not. This means that tea may also assist with weight loss by accelerating the oxidation of fat.

The stimulant in tea, as in coffee, is caffeine. This natural compound activates our nervous system and our metabolic rate, increasing concentration and sensitivity. A cup of tea contains much lower levels of caffeine than coffee: a 7 oz (200 ml) cup of tea contains about 40 mg of caffeine whereas the average cup of instant coffee contains just over 60 mg and a cup of brewed coffee contains as much as 150 mg. Up to 300 mg a day is considered reasonable and safe, whereas 600 mg or more is regarded as excessive and likely to contribute to raised blood pressure and therefore increase the risk of stroke and heart attack.

Tea is often taken after a meal because it aids digestion by helping the breakdown of meats and fats; indeed, after an evening of wine or other alcohol, several cups of tea are always helpful as a pick-me-up. Scientific research also suggests that the chemicals in tea may have the effect of counteracting carcinogens in certain foods, for example fried and grilled meat.

However, as with everything, overdosing on tea can have negative side effects, among them irritable stomach membranes, insomnia, and stained teeth. Such symptoms are normally associated not only with high volumes of intake, but also with particularly strong brews of tea. Generally speaking, any side effects are easily mitigated by drinking lightly brewed tea, and any Chinese doctor or tea connoisseur would certainly say the same.

Introducing the Healing Teas

In China there is a popular household saying that literally translates as "Sickness is cured when it is shallow." Because tea is drunk throughout China all day, every day, and the prevailing expectation is to keep oneself in optimum health, each family will treat minor dips in health with household tea-based cures. Minor ailments will be cured by taking the tea so that there is no need to see a doctor. Only more acute conditions that have not responded to early treatment will be treated professionally. Each of the following recipes is a mild treatment and not an instant cure for the ailments listed. Each tea is taken at the first indication of an imbalance in the body, which if untreated will become an ailment.

The tea recipes that follow are examples of these common treatments. They contain ingredients that are staples in Chinese households. Because of the presence of large Chinese communities in the West, it is now possible to obtain these ingredients from Chinese or Asian stores, or, in the case of unusual dried ingredients, a Chinese herbalist.

Taking the Tea

The effect of taking the tea is mild and cumulative. You should take 2–3 small cups of the tea frequently throughout the day for 2–3 days or until you feel better. Don't take more than 2–3 small cups of the tea at any one time and drink the teas hot, unless otherwise specified. If they should be drunk cold, allow them to cool and then refrigerate. Do not add ice.

If you wish, you may strain the tea when pouring it into a cup, although the Chinese usually allow the solid matter to just settle at the bottom of the pot. You can pour excess liquid from the pot and use the ingredients one more time by adding fresh boiling water. The tea ingredients should not be allowed to stand in the pot for more than 10 hours before being discarded.

It is best to take the tea between meals. When you are eating, try not to drink too much water as the gastric fluid will be diluted and digestion impaired. It is also important not to take strong tea immediately after eating, as it will cause the stomach muscles to contract and you may develop indigestion.

If you find that any of the ingredients are unpalatable, you can weaken the strength by reducing the quantity of that ingredient. For recipes with intensely flavored ingredients you may want to keep a teapot especially for making these teas, or make them in a saucepan. Alternatively, you can halve the ingredients and make them in the large decorative mugs with lids available from Chinese stores. These mugs will hold about 1½ cups (430 ml) of liquid.

When you make the tea, always use the best quality water, such as spring water. If you are using tap water, pass it through a charcoal filter to improve the quality. You can make most of the teas with your own favorite tea and as strong or weak as you prefer.

THE TEAS

FOR SLIMMING
Oolong tea 120

FOR HIGH BLOOD PRESSURE
Banana tea 120
Lotus nut tea 121

FOR REDUCING INTERNAL HEAT
Yellow chrysanthemum tea 122

TONIC TEAS
Peanut and ginger tea 123
Lychee and plum tea 124
Dragon eye tea 124
Dry-fried rice tea 126
Light treasure tea 126

TO STRENGTHEN THE IMMUNE SYSTEM
Shrimp tea 128

TO RESTORE THE BLOOD
Chinese red date tea 128

TO REPLENISH BLOOD CHI
Sesame and mushroom tea 129

FOR THE COMMON COLD
Ginger and spring onion tea 130

FOR COLDS WITH A SLIGHT FEVERISH HEADACHE
Sweet ginger tea 130

FOR COUGHS
White radish tea 131

FOR ITCHY, TICKLY THROAT BUT NO COUGH
Licorice tea 131

FOR DRY SORE THROAT
Honey and lemon tea 132

FOR THROAT INFECTIONS OR SORE GUMS
Sweet tea 132

FOR FLU
Lei Ch'a 133

SUMMER TEAS
Hot chrysanthemum tea 134
Chilled chrysanthemum tea 134
Tomato tea 135

FOR DIARRHEA OR LOOSE BOWELS
Mung bean tea 136

FOR BOWEL PAIN
Rice vinegar tea 136

FOR WEIGHT LOSS

Oolong tea

From its first discovery, tea has been appreciated as an aid to weight loss. All types of tea share this quality but Oolong tea is superior to all others in this respect. The effect of this tea is to reduce fat around the body organs. It can be taken two or three times a day and there will be a gradual loss of weight.

2 rounded teaspoons of Oolong tea
3 cups (850 ml) of water

Boil the water. Rinse the pot with hot water then add the Oolong tea to the empty, heated pot. When the water has reached a fast boil, pour onto the leaves and allow the tea to stand for 2–3 minutes. Pour into a cup and allow to cool very slightly before drinking.

FOR HIGH BLOOD PRESSURE

Banana tea

As we age, it is usual for our blood pressure to rise. High blood pressure can also be a hereditary condition or be caused by too much salt and animal fat in the diet or excessive alcohol consumption.

This tea can be taken daily by anyone over 45 years old or others who are suffering from high blood pressure. As the banana taste is quite strong and will scent the teapot, it is best to use a mug to make this tea, preferably a Chinese mug with a lid.

Banana
Green tea
1½ cups (430 ml) of water

In China, bananas are very small and a whole banana might be used for this recipe. In the West, bananas are very large and you will just need a peeled piece about 1in. (2.5 cm) long for each mug. Peel a banana, cut off and mash a 1-in.-(2.5-cm-) long piece, and put it into the mug. Add green tea to taste. Bring the water to a fast boil and pour over the tea and banana. Cover and leave to stand for 2–3 minutes before drinking.

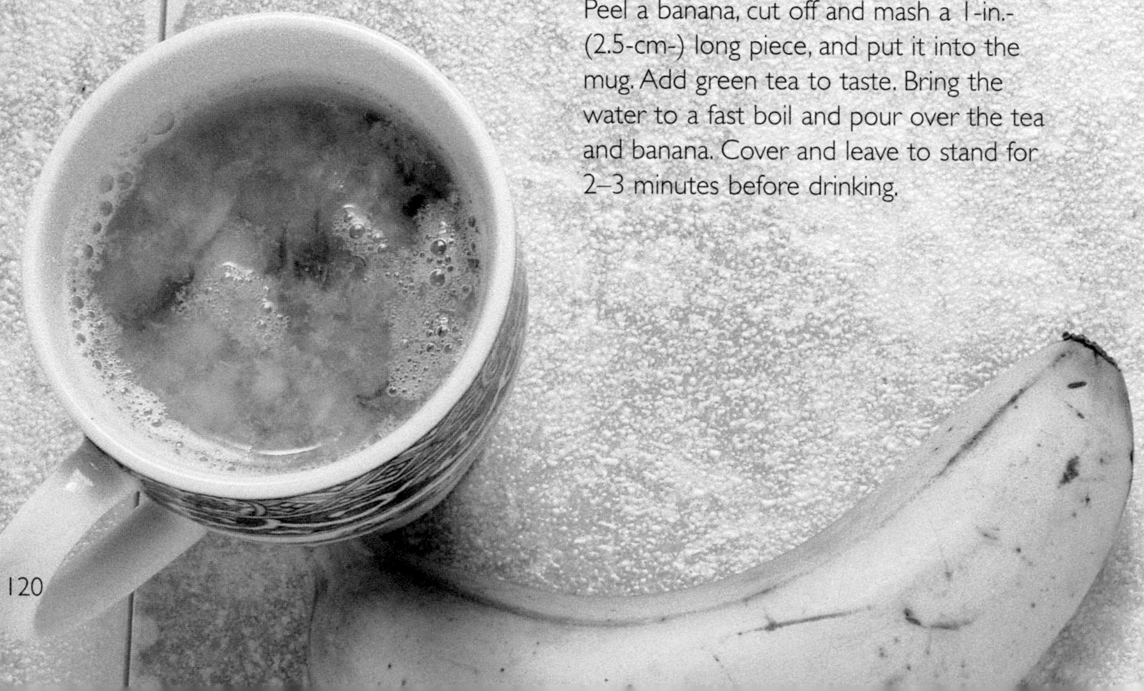

FOR HIGH BLOOD PRESSURE

Lotus nut tea

The lotus nut is the seed of the lotus plant (*Nelumbo nucifera*), which has been a sacred symbol in Buddhism for over 5,000 years. These fat round nuts are found within the round seed pod, which has a flat top with large round holes in it. The nuts look rather like peanuts but have a brown skin. The skin itself has a dry, leathery taste. You can buy lotus nuts in a plastic package in Chinese markets, although make sure you buy ones that still have their skins. The lotus nut is useful for lowering blood pressure.

12–15 lotus nuts
Green tea
3 cups (850 ml) of water

Warm the pot and add 12–15 lotus nuts with green tea to taste. Bring the water to a fast boil and pour it over the tea and nuts. Cover and leave to stand for 5 minutes before drinking.

There is another way to make this tea. Put 12–15 nuts into a saucepan with 3 cups (850 ml) of cold water. Bring the water to the boil and allow to boil for 1–2 minutes. Remove the pan from the heat and add green tea to taste. Leave for a further 1–2 minutes before drinking.

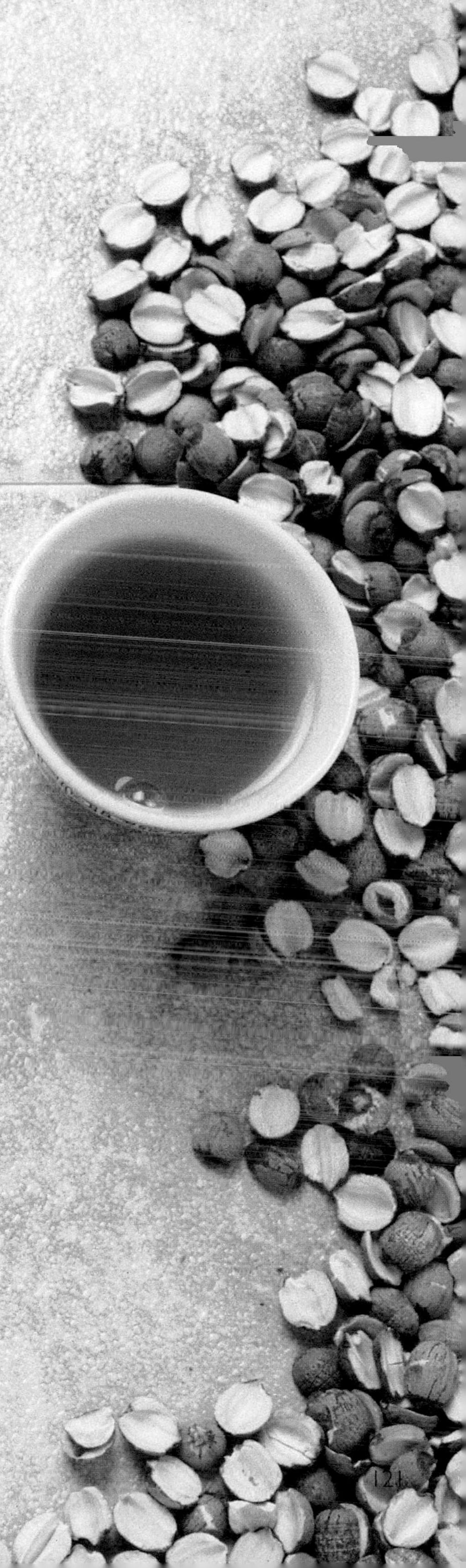

FOR REDUCING INTERNAL HEAT

Yellow chrysanthemum tea

Waking up in the morning with a sticky discharge around your eyes or poor vision is an indication of too much heat in the body. Chrysanthemum tea reduces heat and clears the eyes. You can buy the flowers, dried and in plastic packages, from Chinese markets or herbalists. Be sure to buy yellow chrysanthemums rather than white ones, which are used for treating sunstroke (see p. 134). There are three ways of making this tea with the following ingredients:

10–20 yellow chrysanthemum flowers
3 cups (850 ml) of water

Method one

Set the water to boil and warm the teapot. Add 10–20 flowers to the heated pot. When the water has reached a fast boil pour it over the flowers. Leave to stand for 2–3 minutes before drinking. (You may wish to strain the tea into a cup, as the flowers break up and tend to float.)

Method two

For a fuller taste, brew some tea leaves with the chrysanthemums. To make the tea, add the flowers and the tea of your choice to the pot and proceed as before.

Method three

If you have a sweet tooth you can add rock sugar to this tea. Rock sugar crystals can be bought from Chinese stores. It has a very pleasant taste and is a lovely light golden color. If the lumps of sugar are too large, wrap them in a dish towel or paper and hit them with a hammer or rolling pin to break them into smaller pieces.

Wash and drain the flowers, and put them into a saucepan. Add the water and bring to the boil. Turn the heat down low and continue to cook the flowers for 25 minutes. Add the rock sugar and cook for another 3 minutes. Allow the tea to cool slightly, then strain and drink.

You can use the flowers twice to make tea. The flavor will be weaker the second time, but the tea will retain its curative properties.

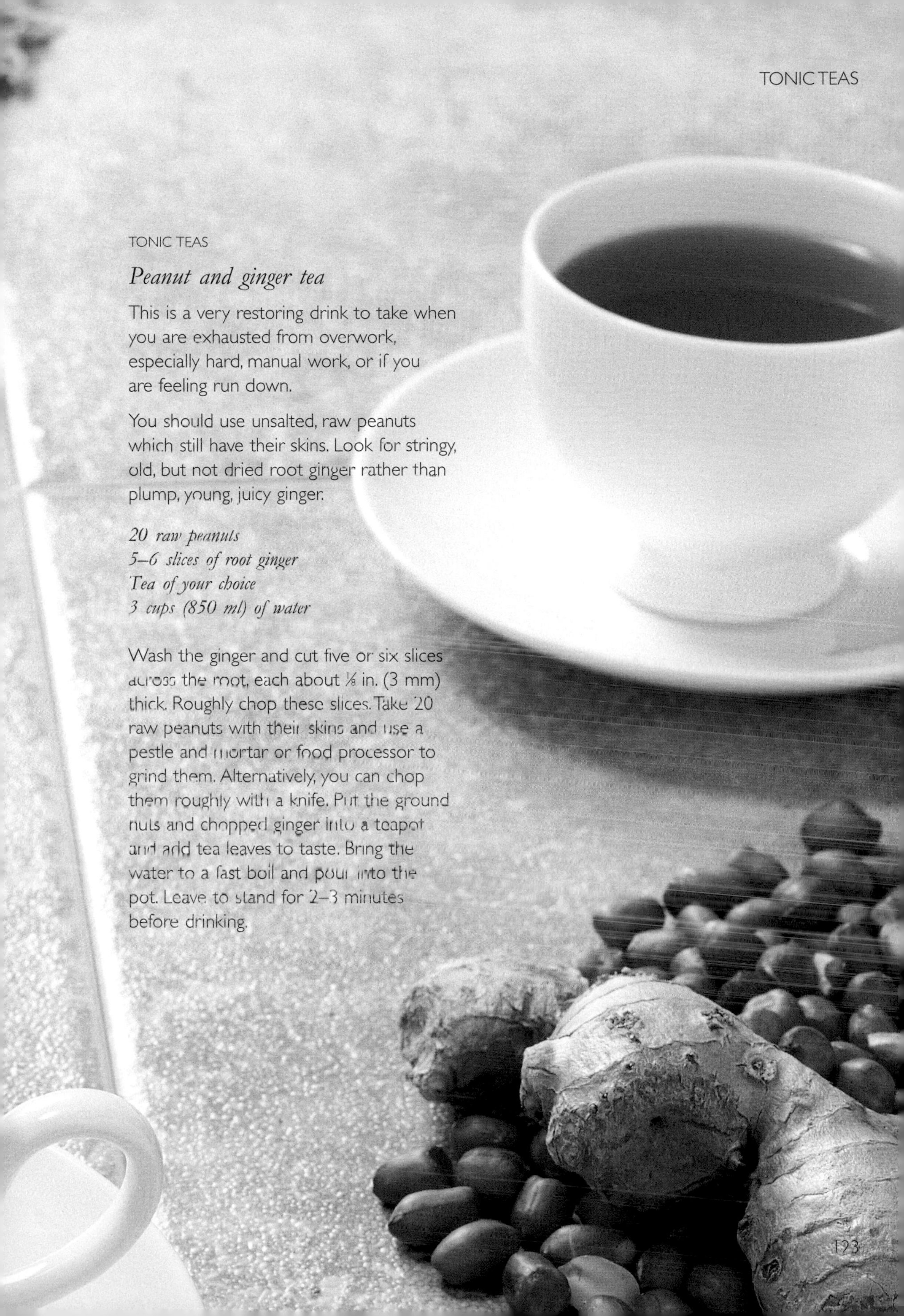

Peanut and ginger tea

This is a very restoring drink to take when you are exhausted from overwork, especially hard, manual work, or if you are feeling run down.

You should use unsalted, raw peanuts which still have their skins. Look for stringy, old, but not dried root ginger rather than plump, young, juicy ginger.

20 raw peanuts
5–6 slices of root ginger
Tea of your choice
3 cups (850 ml) of water

Wash the ginger and cut five or six slices across the root, each about ⅛ in. (3 mm) thick. Roughly chop these slices. Take 20 raw peanuts with their skins and use a pestle and mortar or food processor to grind them. Alternatively, you can chop them roughly with a knife. Put the ground nuts and chopped ginger into a teapot and add tea leaves to taste. Bring the water to a fast boil and pour into the pot. Leave to stand for 2–3 minutes before drinking.

TONIC TEAS

Lychee and plum tea

This delightful fruit tea not only pleases the palate but also boosts energy levels. However, only take the tea twice a week as lychees have very strong yang energy. The plum used is a preserved plum that you will find in Chinese stores, and looks similar to a date. You will also need a fresh lychee and some rock sugar (see p. 122). Lychees are in season from May through August. You can spice up the flavor of the tea by adding a little fresh ginger root.

1 fresh lychee
1 preserved plum
1 small piece rock sugar
1 thin slice ginger root (optional)
1½ cups (430 ml) of water

Cut the plum in half and remove the stone. Peel the lychee and remove the stone. Put the lychee, plum, sugar, and ginger into a large Chinese mug. Fill up the mug with boiling water, stir it quickly, and put on the lid. Leave to stand for 2–3 minutes, stir, and then drink.

If you like, you can try adding a pinch of green tea to freshen the taste. You can also top off your mug with more water and then eat the fruit when you have finished the tea.

Dragon eye tea

Dragon eye is a direct translation of the Mandarin name of this fruit, which is called "longan" in Cantonese. Longan look similar to lychees in size and shape but have smooth pale brown skins. Like lychees, they are in season from May through August. They are highly prized in Chinese medicine, as they help restore blood chi. They can be used fresh or dried. When fresh, the flesh is white; when dried, the skin is a darker brown and the flesh a rich dark brown. The flesh is sweet and fragrant. Whether you use fresh or dried longan always remove the skin.

To prepare the tea, follow the recipe for lychee and plum tea (left), only use a dragon eye instead of the lychee.

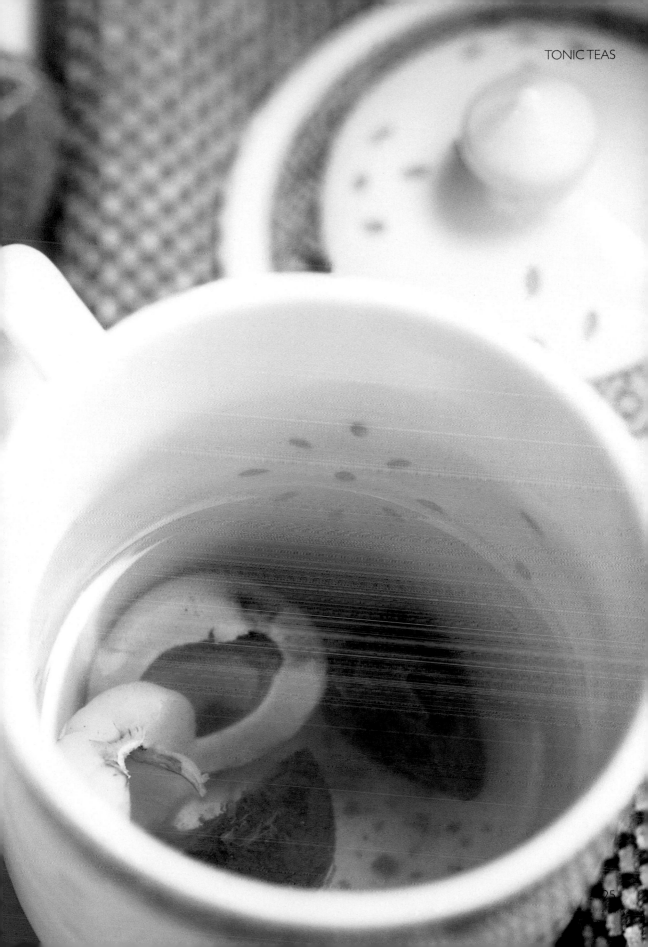

TONIC TEAS

Dry-fried rice tea

This energy-boosting tea has the ability to balance the hot (yang) and cool (yin) energy in the body and is used for people with too much yin who need more yang. It is not recommended for yang people.

It has a good nutty flavor and, once prepared, you can keep the dried ingredients in an airtight jar. In Japan it is so popular that you can buy it ready-mixed.

1 cup of long grain rice
1 cup of green tea leaves
3 cups (850 ml) of water

Heat the wok and tip in the rice. You do not need any oil. Stir-fry the rice until the grains are light golden and smell toasty. Allow the rice to cool and then add the green tea leaves and mix gently.

To make the tea, put five teaspoonfuls of it into the teapot and add boiling water. Allow to stand for 2–3 minutes before drinking. You can refill the teapot with freshly boiled water once or twice.

Eight treasure tea

This very healthy, energy-boosting tea can be taken twice a week. The eight ingredients are the treasures of this recipe. They should all be available from a good Chinese market or herbalist.

Green tea
2 white chrysanthemums
1 small piece of dried mandarin orange peel
1 longan or dragon eye (fresh or dried)
1 red date
1 tiny piece ginseng root
1 dried medlar berry (gou qi zi)
1 piece rock sugar
1 sultana or dried apple slice
1½ cups (430 ml) of water

Put all the ingredients into a large lidded mug and pour over the boiling water. Allow to stand for about 3 minutes before drinking. You can refill your mug with freshly boiled water two or three times.

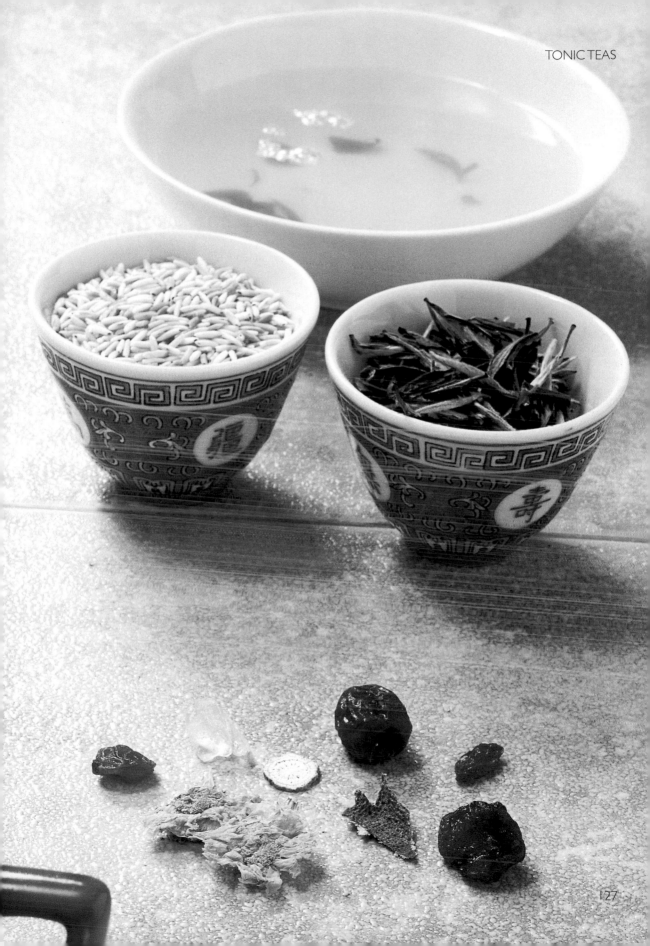

TO STRENGTHEN THE IMMUNE SYSTEM

Shrimp tea

You can buy tiny, pink, dried shrimps in plastic packages from Chinese markets. Avoid any that are grayish-brown, as they will not be fresh. Once you have opened the pack, store it in the fridge.

30 dried shrimps (approximately)
Tea of your choice
3 cups (850 ml) of water

Take about 30 shrimps and rinse them in cold water. Put the shrimps with the tea leaves into a saucepan. Bring some water to the boil and pour over the shrimps and tea. Cover for 2–3 minutes and serve. When you have drunk the tea you may eat the shrimps.

TO RESTORE THE BLOOD

Chinese red date tea

The Chinese red date (Hung Tsao, Da Zao, Da Tsao, jujube, *Ziziphus jujube*) is commonly used in a restorative tea for after childbirth or menstruation, or for anyone who has suffered blood loss.

Red dates are native to China, Japan, India, and Afghanistan and are not like the brown Egyptian sugary dates. They are a very bright red color, small, and oval-shaped with a very shiny, deeply wrinkled skin like a walnut. They taste sweet but not too sweet. You can buy them in Chinese markets in plastic packages. Make sure you remove the stones for this tea (it is sometimes possible to buy stoneless dates).

6–8 Chinese red dates
Tea of your choice
Rock sugar to taste (see p. 122)
3 cups (850 ml) of water

Pick out 6–8 dates and rinse them in cold water. Carefully cut them in half and remove the stone. Put the flesh into a pot with the tea of your choice. Boil the water and pour it over the dates and tea. Add a little rock sugar and allow it to stand for 5 minutes before drinking.

TO REPLENISH BLOOD CHI

Sesame amd mushroom tea

This recipe replenishes blood chi and soft-ens and smoothes the skin. You will need black not golden sesame seeds. Use wood ear dried mushrooms, which are black on one side and beige on the other. Do not confuse them with cloud ear mushrooms, which are much smaller, black on one side, and white on the other. Wood ear mush-rooms are much more nourishing than cloud ears. Wood ear mushrooms and black sesame seeds are available in Chinese markets.

1 small teaspoon black sesame seeds
2-sq.-in. (5-sq.-cm) piece of dried wood ear mushroom
Tea of your choice
3 cups (850 ml) of water

Put the sesame seeds and the piece of wood ear into a mortar and grind them together with a pestle. Alternatively, you can quickly whiz them in a food processor. Put the mixture into a pot and add tea leaves of your choice. Bring the water to the boil and pour it over the ingredients. Leave to stand for 2–3 minutes before drinking. Afterward, you may eat the residue with a spoon.

FOR THE COMMON COLD

Ginger and spring onion tea

Choose old, stringy root ginger rather than a young, juicy piece. Spring onions can be as thin as a pencil or up to 1 in. (2.5 cm) thick. Use one large or two small spring onions.

4–5 slices old ginger root
2 small spring onions, white parts only
Green tea
3 cups (850 ml) of water

Wash the ginger root and cut 4–5 slices, about ⅛ in. (3 mm) thick across the grain. Wash the spring onions and cut off the green leaves — you only need the white parts. Slice the white parts in half lengthwise and put the ginger and spring onion into the teapot with some green tea leaves. Bring the water to the boil and pour it over the ingredients. Cover the pot and leave to stand for 2–3 minutes before drinking.

You can make this tea more potent by adding a little good-quality sea salt.

FOR COLDS WITH SLIGHT FEVERISH HEADACHE

Sweet ginger tea

Choose old, stringy ginger root and golden rock sugar from a Chinese market for this soothing tea. Rock sugar is sold in small boxes. If the lumps are very large, wrap them in a dish towel and break them with a hammer or rolling pin into smaller pieces.

6–7 slices old ginger root
Green tea
Rock sugar
3 cups (850 ml) of water

Wash the ginger root and cut 6–7 slices, about ⅛ in. (3 mm) thick across the grain. Put the ginger root into a teapot with some green tea. Bring the water to the boil, pour it into the pot, and add rock sugar to taste. Stir the tea briefly, then cover the pot. Leave to stand for 2–3 minutes before drinking.

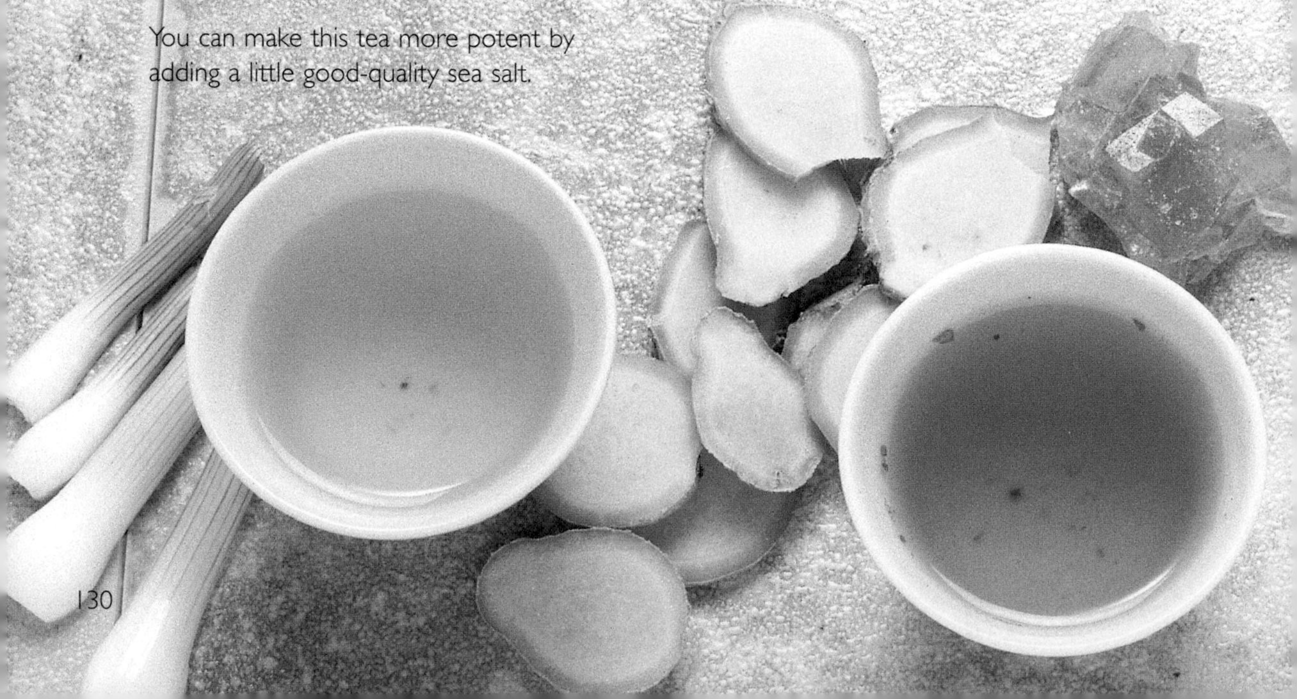

FOR COUGHS

White radish tea

White radishes are often called daikon in Western supermarkets. Use a fresh white radish for this tea. The flavor is quite strong so you will only need to use a small piece. You will also need some good quality sea salt.

1-in.- (2.5-cm-) long piece white radish
Tea of your choice
Sea salt
3 cups (850 ml) of water

Cut and peel a 1-in.- (2.5-cm-) long piece of radish and discard the skin. Roughly chop the radish into small pieces and put it into the teapot with some tea leaves and a little sea salt. Bring the water to the boil and pour it over the ingredients. Cover the pot and leave the tea to stand for 2–3 minutes before drinking.

FOR AN ITCHY, TICKLY THROAT WITH NO COUGH

Licorice tea

Chinese licorice (*Glycyrrhiza uralensis*, or gan cao) tastes good and benefits all the body organs. It is particularly soothing for the lungs and throat. You can buy the thinly sliced dried root in plastic packages in Chinese markets.

6–7 pieces of dried licorice root
Tea of your choice
3 cups (850 ml) of water

Put 6–7 pieces of Chinese licorice into a teapot with some tea leaves of your choice. Bring the water to the boil and pour into the pot. Allow to stand for 5 minutes before drinking.

FOR A DRY SORE THROAT

Honey and lemon tea

Lemon is very good for treating the throat. Honey, or feng mi, must be used with care as it will change its properties if it is heated. It is important to let the tea cool down until it is only lukewarm before adding the honey. People who suffer from chronic loose bowels should add the honey when the tea is still hot.

Half a lemon, preferably organic
Red tea
Honey
3 cups (850 ml) of water

Wash the lemon and cut it in half. Take one half, chop it roughly, and crush it before putting it into the teapot. Add red tea leaves to taste. Bring the water to a fast boil and then pour it over the lemon and tea leaves. Cover the pot and allow it to stand until lukewarm. Add honey to taste and serve.

If you would like to drink this tea hot you can substitute rock sugar for the honey.

Prepare the lemon and put it into a saucepan with the water. Bring it to the boil and add the rock sugar. Reduce the heat and cook for 2 minutes. Take the pan off the heat and add red tea to taste. Allow to stand for 2–3 minutes before drinking.

FOR THROAT INFECTIONS OR SORE GUMS

Sweet tea

This tea is good for throat infections and sore gums. You can also gargle with the tea or use it as a mouthwash.

Green or Oolong tea of your choice
Rock sugar
3 cups (850 ml) of water

To make a strong brew, put 4–5 tea-spoons of tea into the teapot and pour in the boiling water. Add rock sugar to the pot and leave to stand for 2–3 minutes before drinking.

FOR FLU

Lei Ch'a (ground tea)

This very famous tea is used to treat flu or flu-like symptoms. There is a story about this tea, which dates from the Three Kingdoms period (A.D. 221–277).

A famous general was with his army in a mountainous district when he and all of his soldiers fell ill with flu. The local people knew of a special tea to treat the illness, but the recipe was a closely guarded secret. Nonetheless, the villagers decided that they had to try and help the army and gave them the tea to drink. The general and his army recovered and the tea became famous. Today, visitors to mountain villages are sometimes welcomed with this tea.

1 teaspoon green tea leaves
1 dessertspoon of long grain white rice, uncooked
2–3 thin slices of fresh root ginger, cut across the grain
3 cups (850 ml) of water

Wash the rice and finely chop the ginger slices. Put the tea, rice, and ginger into a mortar with a little cold water and use a pestle to grind them into a fine paste (you may also use a food processor).

Pour the water into a saucepan and bring it to the boil. Add the paste and continue to boil, stirring clockwise for 1–2 minutes. Remove from heat and allow to cool slightly before drinking.

You may adjust the proportions of the ingredients to taste.

SUMMER TEAS

In summer, when it is very hot, people run the risk of getting sunstroke. Cooling teas can help prevent and treat mild sunstroke. They also quench thirst and improve the appetite. Dried white chrysanthemum flowers are especially useful for this.

Hot chrysanthemum tea

This white chrysanthemum tea is good for treating mild sunstroke.

20 dried white chrysanthemum flowers
Light green or green tea
3 cups (850 ml) of water

Wash the chrysanthemum flowers and put them into a pot and add some light green or green tea. Bring the water to the boil and pour into the pot. Cover and allow to stand for 2–3 minutes before drinking.

Chilled chrysanthemum tea

This variation is an ideal drink for hot summer parties. As well as helping to prevent sunstroke it is also an excellent thirst quencher. Big soup tureens, heat-resistant bowls, and large jugs are all ideal vessels for serving this tea.

Half a package of dried white chrysanthemum flowers
7–8 pints (4–4½ liters) of water
Honey or rock sugar to taste

Wash the chrysanthemum flowers and put them into a large saucepan with the water. Bring it to the boil, reduce the heat, and continue to cook for half an hour. If you wish to use rock sugar add it at this stage. Remove the pan from the heat, allow to cool slightly, and strain the tea into the tureen or bowl. Allow the tea to cool completely and chill in the refrigerator before serving.

If you use honey, cover the pot and wait until the tea is lukewarm before adding it.

Tomato tea

In the summer when it is very hot it is all too easy to lose your appetite. This tea will perk up your appetite. If you like, you can sweeten the tea with a little sugar.

1 tomato (about the size of a ping pong ball)
Green tea
3 cups (850 ml) of water
Sugar (optional)

Wash the tomato, but do not peel it. Roughly dice the tomato and put it into a pot with some green tea leaves. Bring the water to the boil and pour into the pot. Add sugar to taste, cover, and leave to stand for 2–3 minutes before drinking.

FOR DIARRHEA OR LOOSE BOWELS

Mung bean tea

Mung beans are small beans with green skins and yellow flesh. Whole mung beans can be sprouted and the sprouts used in stir-fries. Split mung beans without their skins can be used whole or ground into a fine flour. For this recipe buy pale yellow mung bean flour from Asian stores, or grind your own with a pestle and mortar or in a spice or coffee grinder. It is important to use white sugar for this recipe.

Tea of your choice
1 teaspoon mung bean flour
3 cups (850 ml) of water
White sugar to taste

Put some tea of your choice into a pot with a teaspoon of mung bean flour. Bring the water to the boil and pour into the pot. Add a little sugar if you wish, cover, and leave to stand for 2–3 minutes before drinking.

FOR BOWEL PAIN

Rice vinegar tea

This is a very effective tea for relieving pain in the lower bowel. You will need white rice vinegar, which you can buy in Chinese markets.

3–4 teaspoons white rice vinegar
Green tea
3 cups (850 ml) of water

Put some green tea into a teapot. Bring the water to the boil and pour into the pot. Add 3–4 teaspoons of vinegar and allow to stand for 2–3 minutes before drinking.

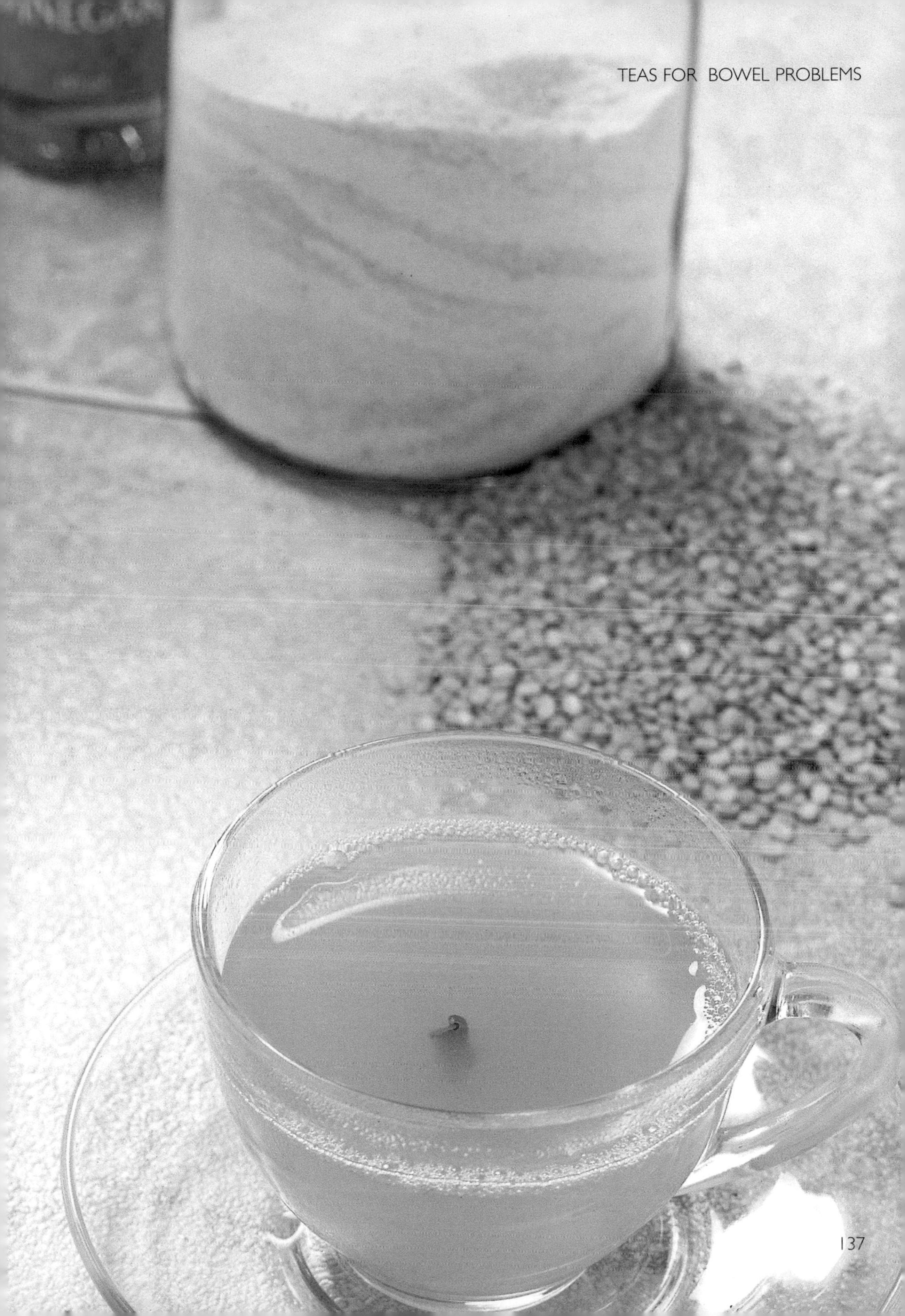

Cautions and Uses of Tea

Don't drink

Scalding hot tea, for obvious reasons.

Cold tea, as it spoils the digestion.

Tea before before eating in the morning.

Very strong tea, unless it is a special medicinal brew.

Tea that has been left to grow cold in the pot. It will be stewed, strong, and bitter.

Tea that has been left overnight and reheated. However, don't throw it away, as it has many other uses (see opposite).

Tea that has been made with dirty water or water polluted with chemicals.

Poor-quality tea. Just as a wine connoisseur will pick the finest wine he can afford to buy, splurge and buy quality tea. Cheap tea is likely to be of poor quality and badly made. This will be apparent in the taste.

Badly stored tea. If it is damp, it will have deteriorated and have a musty smell. Tea should be so dry that it has a rustling sound when shaken. It should always smell good: a bitter tea should smell bitter, a fragrant tea fragrant, and so on.

Tea after eating lamb. Even though the lamb was tender, the tea will toughen it in the stomach and slow down its progress through the bowel, causing constipation.

Tea for one hour before or after taking medicine of any kind, Western or Chinese.

When not to drink tea

Children under two years of age should not drink tea because it interferes with the body's ability to absorb iron and can cause anemia. Similarly, too much tea taken during pregnancy is unhealthy for mother and fetus. A little weak tea is fine.

People who have a weak constitution or delicate stomach should avoid taking tea, as it can damage the stomach lining and interfere with the absorption of nutrients.

Tea drunk on an empty, delicate stomach can cause nausea, stomach pains, and vomiting.

Too much tea can stress the kidneys. Tea is a diuretic and will cause excessive urination and, consequently, dehydration. Normally, a cup of tea will take five to six hours to pass through the body organs. If the kidney is stressed or unhealthy, then its course will be more rapid — two to three hours. Particularly in these cases, the kidneys need rest, so people with delicate kidneys should not take tea before going to bed. Also, the slight caffeine content may keep them awake.

Older people and sick people, especially diabetics, should not take tea before going to bed. A glass of water or a hot milky drink is best. They should not drink strong tea either.

Sufferers of high blood pressure should not drink strong tea as it increases the heart rate and strains the kidneys.

Women taking birth control pills should not drink strong tea.

During menstruation, tea can increase blood flow.

People suffering from stress should not take tea. It will not calm them and will exaggerate their symptoms.

If you have important deadlines to meet and think that drinking tea will keep you awake, it may, but expect to feel more tired the next day.

Tea contracts the stomach muscles so too much tea before a meal will spoil your appetite.

Anyone who has intestinal ulcers should avoid tea because of its slight acidity.

Anyone taking a ginseng treatment or other potent medicine should not drink tea for 24 hours. Strong tea can interfere with the subtle properties of many medicines.

Uses for tea

As a mouthwash after eating

If you bite your tongue while eating, have a mouth infection, or sore throat, warm strong tea will both cleanse and promote healing.

Tea can also be used externally as an antibiotic and cleanser.

To disinfect cuts before applying first aid.

For eye infections — steam from a hot cup of tea or an eyebath of lukewarm tea.

For smelly feet. Soak feet in old warm tea for 10 minutes and then dry carefully before retiring to bed.

If you have been handling fish and your skin smells fishy, carefully wash your hands in strong tea — Oolong works best.

If you are allergic to detergent you can use tea to clean crockery.

To soothe infected skin, make up a bag of tea to use in the bath. Choose a green tea or a fragrant flower tea.

A little bag of used, dried tea leaves will absorb smells in the refrigerator.

Collect and dry old tea leaves to make a little pillow to promote calmness and sleep

To clean windows and mirrors use a cheap tea.

To keep mosquitoes away use the smoke from burning tea leaves.

To enhance the flavor of boiled eggs, add a little tea to the water.

To make a very good acidic compost, recycle your tea leaves in the garden.

About the Authors

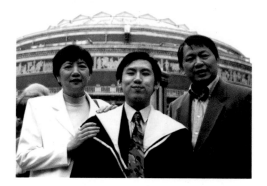

Born in 1948 in Hong Kong, Master Lam Kam Chuen is a preserver and practitioner of more than one form of Chinese cultural heritage. He is a recognized master of the arts of Tai Chi and Chi Kung, a practitioner of a special osteopathy-like branch of Traditional Chinese medicine, and a master of Feng Shui.

In 1976 he came to the West and settled in the United Kingdom where he became the first Tai Chi instructor appointed to teach in the Inner London Education Authority. However, his teaching was not limited to Tai Chi and in 1987 he gave the first European demonstration of the art of Zhan Zhuang Chi Kung. Later, he taught and practiced medicine at The Lam Clinic in London's Chinatown. Now, his practice is near Waterloo station.

Following the widely acclaimed TV series *The Way of the Warrior*, Master Lam was invited to act as consultant to the sequel publication, *The Way of Harmony* (later renamed *The Book of Soft Martial Arts*). Following that, his first ground-breaking publication by Gaia Books, *The Way of Energy*, was launched in 1991, introducing the system of Zhan Zhuang Chi Kung. This was followed by *Step-by-Step Tai Chi* and *The Way of Healing*.

Television viewers in Britain will find Master Lam familiar via the TV series *Stand Still — Be Fit*, which was broadcast on Channel 4 in 1995 and is now available on video under the same title.

Master Lam has also studied Feng Shui extensively under four masters in Hong Kong and Taiwan, each of whom is an acknowledged master in specialized aspects of Feng Shui. It was only relatively recently that Master Lam practiced the art publicly, as it gained recognition in communities beyond the Chinese. Partly due to his concern with the art being preserved in the correct form,

Master Lam was persuaded to create *The Feng Shui Handbook: How to Create a Healthier Living and Working Environment*. Its sequels were *The Personal Feng Shui Manual* and *The Feng Shui Kitchen* — the latter was co-produced with his wife, Kai Sin.

Master Lam and his wife first met as young teenagers while studying martial arts. They married in the early 1970s and had three sons, who grew up in an environment of cultural heritage. Gaia Books, knowing that Master Lam and his family practice the traditional Chinese style of living, asked Master Lam to write a book about the art of drinking tea. Thus, together with his wife and their second son, Tin Yu, this work was produced. *The Way of Tea* is the result of a family collaboration, combining Master Lam's healing expertise, Kai Sin's knowledge of domestic tradition, and Tin Yu's deep understanding of the Chinese way of life.

Consultations and advice
Anyone who would like an individual consultation with Master Lam may contact him at:

The Lam Association
1 Hercules Road, London SE1 7DP, UK.
Tel/fax +44 (0) 20 7261 9049
Mobile +44 (0)7831 802598

For general information visit Master Lam's website at: www.lamassociation.org

Author's Acknowledgments

It is common knowledge throughout the world that we Chinese are a tea-drinking culture, but to have the chance to celebrate this part of our heritage is rare indeed. We are delighted and indebted to those who created this opportunity.

During the course of producing this book we have relearnt forgotten knowledge and found a new depth of appreciation for each cup of tea we drink. We value the intensity of the work and the level of craftsmanship manifested in this wonderful drink. We offer our thanks and respect to everyone in the tea industry for all the delicious teas our family has drunk over the years.

I, LAM Kam Chuen, would also like to express my deepest gratitude to my wife, Kai Sin, not just for her partnership in the making of this book, but also for her caring support, which has given me, and our sons, a healthy and pleasant lifestyle. She has created in us all a deep respect for the food we eat and the nourishment it gives us. I owe much to her.

My sons, Tin Yun, Tin Yu and Tin Hun have worked hard to learn Chinese values and wisdom in a Western world, to try to gain the best from both worlds, and to inherit my knowledge. They have on many occasions provided a bridge for me to bring Eastern knowledge to Western understanding. I am in particular debt to my second son, Tin Yu, for working on this project with us. He has recently completed his MSc in Finance at Imperial College, London and has sacrificed much of his post-degree break to work on this book.

We would like to express our gratitude to all the staff of Gaia Books, particularly to Joss Pearson, the Managing Director, who invited us to write The Way of Tea. The book would have been a lifeless collection of text but for the marvellous devotion of Bridget Morley, who poured her expertise into the design.

Pip Morgan has been of great service in the fine-tuning of the text. We hope there will be more opportunities to work together.

Finally, we thank all our relatives and friends, the students of Master Lam and everyone who has worked hard to bring this project to fruition.

Publisher's Acknowledgments

Gaia Books would like to thank Master Lam, Kai Sin, and Tin Yu for sharing with us their knowledge and experience of the "way of tea." We also thank them for their unfailing kindness, enthusiasm, and hospitality. Thanks also to Mr. Edward Bramah of the Bramah Museum of Tea and Coffee, London; Gina Douglas, Librarian of the Linnaean Society of London; Susanna Abbott; William Revell; Sam Scott-Hunter; and Kate Rushforth.

PHOTO CREDITS

A

afternoon tea 32, 33
America 17, 33, 36, 37
annual tea production worldwide 17
antioxidants 117
Assam 17, 30, 34

B

baking the tea 47
Bedford, Duchess of 33
"big bowl tea" 22, 90
black tea 11, 40, 42, 68–69
    He Lung Chu 68
    Wu Tang 69, 69
Blechynden, Richard 17, 37
Bodhidharma 15
Book of Tea, The 26
Boston Tea Party 33, 36, 36
British East India Company 17, 30, 32,
    33, 34, 36, 37
Bruce, Major Robert 17, 30
Buddhism 58
Buddhist monk 17, 18, 24
    Dengyo Daishi 17, 24
    Yesai 17

C

caffeine 117
Camellia sinensis 9, 40, 40, 41
cancer 116
Canton 21, 36, 45
carcinogens 117
Catherine of Braganza 33
Ceylon 17
ch'a 5, 14, 24
Ch'a Ching 16, 17, 18
cha do 24, 26
chinaware 17, 20, 36
Chinese dynasties
    Ching 17, 21, 47, 58, 66, 75
    Han 9, 16, 17
    Ming 17, 20, 60, 76, 80, 81
    Sung 16, 17, 20, 29, 44, 45, 46
    Tang 12, 16, 17, 19, 24, 26, 44, 56, 64
    Three Kingdoms 16, 17, 25
    Yüan 47
Chinese emperors
    Chien Lung 58

Huang Ti 14, 15
Hui Tsung 20
Kin Lung 75–76
Shên Nung 14, 17
Tang 18
Chinese medicine 114, 116
cholesterol 117
coffee 17, 117

D

Darjeeling 34, 67
"daughter-in-law tea" 23
dim sum 21, 22, 115
dragon balls 49, 54, 68
dragon eye 124, 126, 126–127
dried red date 23, 113, 126, 128, 128
Dutch East India Company 17, 30

E

England 17, 33

F

fermented tea 40, 47
fire 77
    Men For 77
    Wu For 77
flower teas 70–71, 79
    golden lotus 71
    jasmine 70, 71
    lychee 71
    rose congou 70
fluoride 116
Fortnum and Mason 33
France 32
Fukien 21, 24, 41, 66, 92

G

Germany 32
Golden Age of Tea 16, 17, 20, 45
green tea 11, 33, 40, 42, 62–65, 70, 79
    Ho Chin 63
    Jade Ring 65
    Lo Chu Ch'a 65
    Pi Mo Houn 63
    Polee 45, 64, 64, 78, 84
    Yu Ch'ien Lung Ching 62, 64
Grinding the Tea 44, 46

H

Harrods 33
healing teas 118–137
    banana tea 120, 120
    chilled chrysanthemum tea 134, 135
    Chinese red date tea 128, 128
    ginger and spring onion tea 130, 130
    dragon eye tea 124
    dry-fried rice tea 126, 127
    eight treasure tea 126, 126
    honey and lemon tea 132, 132
    hot chrysanthemum tea 134
    Lei Ch'a 133, 133
    licorice tea 131, 131
    lotus nut tea 121, 121
    lychee and plum tea 124, 125
    mung bean tea 136, 136
    Oolong tea 120
    peanut and ginger tea 123, 123
    rice vinegar tea 136, 137
    sesame and mushroom tea 129, 129
    shrimp tea 128, 128
    sweet ginger tea 130, 130
    sweet tea 132
    tomato tea 135, 135
    white radish tea 131, 131
    yellow chrysanthemum tea 122, 122
Holland 17, 32
Hong Kong 31, 33, 114

I

iced tea 17, 37
India 17, 30, 32, 35, 67
Indonesia 17, 30

J

Jacobson, J. I. L. L. 17, 30
Japan 17, 24, 26, 27, 31
Japanese tea ceremony 24, 26, 27
Jixing sand pottery 20, 81, 83, 85, 92,
    92–111

K

Kenya 17
Killing Green 50, 51, 56
Korea 25, 26
Kung Fu tea 92–111, 92-111
    foot water 100

making the second brew 107
making the tea 103
pouring the tea 104
serving the tea 108
showing the tea 97
using a bowl set 110
washing the cups 95
washing the pot 93
washing the tea 99
Kung Fu tea sets 85, 92–111

L
light green tea 11, 40, 58–61, 79
    Hao Seng 59
    Kwai Shui Kam 61
    Oolong 60, 60, 79
    Ta Hung P'ao 60, 61
    T'ieh Kuan-yin 58, 59, 60, 78, 84,
        97
London 30, 32, 34, 34
loose tea 20, 45, 47, 50
lotus nut 23, 121
Lo Yu 16, 17, 18, 52, 74

M
Malaysia 28
metallic chi 79
modern medical research
    116–117
Mongolia 28, 29
monkey-picked tea 52, 58
    Yang Hsien Yun Wu 52
Muslim 18

N
New York 17, 36

O
Oolong tea 10, 60, 78
    cold top Oolong 41, 60
organic tea 11

P
People's Republic of China 17, 21,
    23, 23
plucking tea 41, 42, 43, 46
Portugal 17, 32

R
red tea 11, 30, 33, 40, 66–67, 70,
    78

Red Keemun 66
Nilgiri 67, 67
Darjeeling 67, 67
Russia 17, 28, 29
    Tsar Alexis 17, 28

S
samovar 29
semi-fermented tea 40, 47, 50, 51
Smacking the Tea 44
Squeezing the Tea 46
Sri Lanka 17, 30
Steaming the Tea 44, 46
Stir-frying Green 48, 50, 51, 56
storing tea leaves 88, 89
Su Yu Ch'a 26, 28
Sullivan, Thomas 17
Swinging Green 47

T
Ta Kuan Ch'a Lun 20
Taiwan 17
tea
    auction 31, 32
    bag 11, 17
    balls 20, 44, 45, 15, 46, 47, 64
    bricks 20, 44, 45, 46, 47, 64
    bowls 91, 91
        Japanese 27
    cautions 138–139
    clipper 37
    gardens 34, 34
    gifts 22–23
    houses 21, 26
    needle 92, 104
    powder 26, 46
    processing 44–51, 48–49
    scoop 92, 91
    tax 20
    tongs 92, 95, 101, 101
Tea Act 36
tea-drinking customs 21, 22–23
teaism 26
tea plants 40–41
    Assam 40
    Cambodia 40
    China 40
    flags 42, 46
    spear 42, 46
teapots 20, 80–87
    choosing 81–82

Malaysian 28
materials for 80
Ming 80, 81
parts of 87, 87
porcelain 17, 20
preparing 84
preserving 86
Tibetan 28
Thailand 28
Tibet 26, 28, 56
types of tea 11, 40, 47–71

U
unfermented tea 47
uses for tea 139

W
water 74–79
    distilled 76
    hard 76
    hot spring 76
    mineral 76
    mountain 74, 75
    quality 74–76
    soft 76
    tap 76
water temperature 77–79
    Chi Pien 78
    crab-eye water 78, 78
    fish-eye water 77, 79
    Hsing Pien 78
    old man water 77, 79
    Sheng Pien 78
    yin-yang 78
ways of drinking tea 21
white tea 11, 20, 10, 11, 53–55
    Pai Hao Yin Chin 54
    Pai Loong Chu 54
    Pai Mu Tan 54
wok 44, 48, 50

Y
Yale, Elihu 33
Yellow Emperor's Classic of Internal
    Medicine, The 14, 15
yellow tea 11, 40, 46, 53, 56–57
    Chün Shan Yin Chin 56, 57

Z
Zen Buddhism 15, 24, 26